# SERIOUS EMOTIONAL DISTURBANCE IN CHILDREN AND ADOLESCENTS

# SERIOUS EMOTIONAL DISTURBANCE IN CHILDREN AND ADOLESCENTS

## Multisystemic Therapy

Scott W. Henggeler
Sonja K. Schoenwald
Melisa D. Rowland
Phillippe B. Cunningham

THE GUILFORD PRESS
New York     London

**Library of Congress Cataloging-in-Publication Data**

Serious emotional disturbance in children and adolescents :
multisystemic therapy / Scott W. Henggeler . . . [et al.].
        p. cm.
Includes bibliographical references and index.
  ISBN 1-57230-780-3
  1. Affective disorders in children. 2. Adolescent psychopathology.
I. Henggeler, Scott W., 1950–
RJ506.D4 S47 2002
618.92′8527—dc21

                                                  2002005009

# About the Authors

**Scott W. Henggeler, PhD,** is Professor in the Department of Psychiatry and Behavioral Sciences at the Medical University of South Carolina and Director of the Family Services Research Center. The Center has recently received the Annie E. Casey Families Count Award as well as the Points of Light Foundation President's Award in recognition of excellence in community service directed at solving community problems. Dr. Henggeler has published approximately 200 journal articles, book chapters, and books; is on the editorial boards of nine journals; and has received grants from the National Institute of Mental Health, the National Institute on Drug Abuse, the National Institute on Alcohol Abuse and Alcoholism, the Office of Juvenile Justice and Delinquency Prevention, the Annie E. Casey Foundation, and others. Dr. Henggeler's research and social policy interests include the development and validation of innovative methods of mental health and substance abuse services for disadvantaged children and their families, as well as efforts for redistributing mental health resources to services that are clinically and cost effective and that preserve family integrity.

**Sonja K. Schoenwald, PhD,** is Associate Professor in the Department of Psychiatry and Behavioral Sciences at the Medical University of South Carolina and Associate Director of the Family Services Research Center. Her current research focuses on the empirical validation, transportability, and dissemination of clinically and cost-effective mental health services for youths with complex problems and their families. Dr. Schoenwald has taken a leadership role in developing the clinical training and quality assurance protocols used to transport multisystemic therapy to community-based sites and in research on the effectiveness of such protocols.

She is also participating in the development of foundation- and state-sponsored initiatives to increase and examine the use of evidence-based practices for children and families in community settings. Dr. Schoenwald has published numerous articles and book chapters and serves on the editorial boards of several journals.

**Melisa D. Rowland, MD,** is Assistant Professor in the Department of Psychiatry and Behavioral Sciences at the Medical University of South Carolina and Medical Director of the Family Services Research Center. Much of Dr. Rowland's research involves developing, implementing, and evaluating clinically effective, family-based interventions for youths presenting with serious emotional and behavioral problems. Currently, she is the primary investigator for a National Institute on Drug Abuse–funded K–12 award focusing on the development of empirically grounded, community-based treatments for youths presenting with substance use disorders. She also serves as coinvestigator for an Annie E. Casey Foundation-funded research evaluation of the clinical and cost effectiveness of a multisystemic therapy (MST)-based continuum of services provided to a population of youths at risk for out-of-home placement due to severe emotional and behavioral problems. Dr. Rowland recently served as project coordinator of a large National Institute of Mental Health-funded R01 clinical trial in which youth in psychiatric crises were randomly assigned to MST family preservation or psychiatric hospitalization. This evaluation of MST for youth with serious emotional disturbance played a central role in the development of the interventions outlined in this text.

**Phillippe B. Cunningham, PhD,** is Associate Professor in the Department of Psychiatry and Behavioral Sciences at the Medical University of South Carolina and Assistant Director of Training of Multisystemic Therapy at the Family Services Research Center. In his current position, Dr. Cunningham supervises family therapists providing intensive family- and home-based services to substance-abusing juvenile delinquents and youths presenting with severe mental health problems. His research interests include (1) issues pertinent to ethnic minority communities, especially community violence and its role in the etiology of antisocial behavior and anxiety disorders (e.g., posttraumatic stress disorder); (2) evaluating innovative and culturally competent clinical services for disadvantaged youths and families, especially community-based services; (3) developing and evaluating community- and school-based violence prevention and intervention strategies; and (4) training and supervising mental health professionals in providing innovative child-centered and family-based services.

# Preface

Every day in every community in the United States, the parents of a child with serious emotional disturbance grapple with the challenges of charting a successful life course for that child. Likewise, every day in every community in the United States, mental health professionals who have dedicated their lives to the cause of children and families grapple with the same challenges. The challenges are particularly great because so little of what is available in the way of treatment and service for children and families can effectively alter the life course of such a child. Thus, the hard work and dedication exhibited by mental health professionals, parents, and children are rarely rewarded with positive outcomes. An effective multisystemic therapy (MST) program can alter the life course of the child with serious emotional disturbance, his or her family, and, potentially, the clinician.

The development of this book was prompted by our experiences in adapting MST to the needs of children and adolescents with serious mental health problems and their families. Although MST has enjoyed widespread success as an effective treatment for adolescents with serious antisocial behavior, many of whom have had co-occurring mental health problems, MST clinical trials and MST programs had never focused specifically on youths with challenging mental health problems. In 1994, however, the National Institute of Mental Health funded a study to examine the effectiveness of MST as an alternative to psychiatric hospitalization of youths with mental health emergencies (i.e., suicidal, homicidal, psychotic). Experiences conducting this study and in other venues have given us great appreciation for the challenges and strengths presented by children with serious emotional disturbance and their fami-

lies. The overarching purpose of this book is to describe the implementation of MST with these children and adolescents and their families.

Helping families to change the life course of children with serious
emotional disturbance requires considerable support for both the family
and the MST practitioner. Regarding the former, MST emphasizes the
explicit development of indigenous support systems (e.g., extended family, neighbors, friends, church members) to provide families with the resources and strategies they need to weather times of stress and crisis.
Similarly, MST programs surround practitioners with considerable emotional and clinical support (e.g., therapists work in teams with strong
supervisory support and ongoing access to expert consultation) to help
achieve favorable outcomes for their clients. No single therapist, no
matter how talented, can be expected to effectively address the broad
range of challenging problems presented by families of children with
serious emotional disturbance. Practitioners deserve access to the
resources needed to accomplish their families' goals. This book assumes
that they have access to these resources. With resources and effective
clinical tools, practitioners can help to change the life trajectories of
these children and their families.

# Acknowledgments

This book is dedicated to the children we continue to love the most, and especially to Sterling, the most recent and imposing addition to the clan. Waylon, Santos, Phillippe, Noelle, Lee, and Jay nevertheless continue to amaze us with their talents, humor, and capacity to humble their "expert" parents.

We thank the many families who have enabled us to pursue this work and greatly appreciate the funding sources that have expedited our research, including the National Institute of Mental Health, the National Institute on Drug Abuse, the National Institute on Alcohol Abuse and Alcoholism, the Annie E. Casey Foundation, and the Office of Juvenile Justice and Delinquency Prevention.

# Contents

**PART I. Essential Clinical Processes**      1

CHAPTER 1.   Introduction to Multisystemic Therapy      3

CHAPTER 2.   MST Principles and Process      17

CHAPTER 3.   Family Interventions and Building Indigenous      38
Family Supports

CHAPTER 4.   Social System Interventions: Service System,      75
School, and Peer

**PART II. Adapting MST to Treat Youths**      97
**with Serious Emotional Disturbance**

CHAPTER 5.   Addressing Psychiatric Emergencies:      99
Staffing, Assessment, and Intervention Protocols
*with Susan G. Pickrel*

CHAPTER 6.   MST-Based Continuum of Care      139

CHAPTER 7.   Case Examples      169

**PART III. Outcomes, Ongoing Research,**                    203
**and Program Development**

CHAPTER 8.   MST Outcomes and Ongoing Research              205

CHAPTER 9.   MST Quality Assurance: Promoting Effective     227
             Implementation in the Field

References                                                  241

Index                                                       256

# PART I

# Essential Clinical Processes

This part presents the core components of multisystemic therapy (MST)—features that do not vary substantively for youths presenting mental health problems, criminal behavior, or substance abuse. These features pertain to the guiding principles of MST; the development and implementation of intervention strategies across individual, family, peer, school, and social systems; and the ongoing tracking of clinical outcomes. Chapters in Part II delineate adaptations of the model that have been made to treat youths with serious emotional disturbance and their families.

# CHAPTER 1

# Introduction to Multisystemic Therapy

Although MST has a well-established track record in treating serious antisocial behavior in adolescents, the model has only recently been adapted to treat serious emotional disturbance in children and adolescents. This chapter describes key bases to the success that MST has achieved in treating adolescent antisocial behavior and suggests that these bases are equally applicable to the effective treatment of serious emotional disturbance in children and adolescents. Moreover, these emphases are consistent with conclusions from the U.S. Surgeon General's Report on Children and Mental Health (U.S. Department of Health and Human Services, [DHHS], 1999), as well as with extant research on the nature of serious emotional disturbance in children and adolescents.

MST is a family- and community-based treatment model that was originally developed in the late 1970s to address the mental health needs of juvenile offenders. Currently, MST is best known for its success in reducing long-term rates of rearrest and out-of-home placement for violent and chronic juvenile offenders. For example, MST is featured in Dr. Delbert Elliott's prestigious Blueprint Series (Elliott, 1998), has been described favorably by respected reviewers in the field of juvenile justice (e.g., Farrington & Welsh, 1999; Tate, Reppucci, & Mulvey, 1995), and was the focus of a bulletin published by the Office of Juvenile Justice and Delinquency Prevention (Henggeler, 1997a).

The success of MST with violent and chronic juvenile offenders and their families led to funding in 1994 from the National Institute of Mental Health (NIMH) to determine whether MST could be adapted to meet the clinical needs of youths presenting psychiatric crises (e.g., suicidal, homicidal, psychotic). In turn, the subsequent success of MST as an alternative to emergency psychiatric hospitalization (see outcomes described in Chapter 8) has led to the development and evaluation of an MST-based continuum of care that addresses the mental health needs of the most challenging child and adolescent clients in communities.

The purpose of this volume is to describe the application of MST to youths with serious emotional disturbance and their families. Much of what is central to the implementation of MST in treating serious antisocial behavior (Henggeler, Schoenwald, Borduin, Rowland, & Cunningham, 1998) also pertains to the treatment of serious emotional disturbance (see Chapters 2–4). Nevertheless, our experience with youths presenting serious mental health problems led to significant adaptations of the model for this deep-end mental health population. These adaptations are detailed in Chapters 5–6; Chapter 7 presents three extended case examples that integrate the invariant features of MST with the more recent adaptations.

Before detailing MST clinical and quality assurance protocols for treating youths with serious emotional disturbance, summarizing the bases for the success of MST is valuable on conceptual and policy levels. Though logical and founded on the existing research literature, these bases generally conflict with the vast majority of prevailing mental health practices. The gap between MST treatment protocols, quality assurance protocols, and models of service delivery and current mental health practices presents substantive barriers to the adoption of MST programs (see Chapter 8) at multiple levels (e.g., therapist, agency, funding structures). Nevertheless, the bases of the success of MST have implications for the broader field of mental health services, irrespective of MST. That is, incorporating any one or some combination of the following bases would likely improve the outcomes associated with prevailing mental health practices.

## BASES OF MST SUCCESS

MST has been identified as a highly promising treatment model by reviewers in the fields of child and adolescent mental health (e.g., Kazdin

& Weisz, 1998; DHHS, 1999), adolescent violence (e.g., Elliott, 1998; Farrington & Welsh, 1999; Tate et al., 1995), and substance abuse (e.g., McBride, VanderWaal, Terry, & VanBuren, 1999; National Institute on Drug Abuse [NIDA], 1999; Stanton & Shadish, 1997). Several features of MST and MST programs account for this promise.

## MST Addresses Risk Factors, Builds Protective Factors

If a problem is multidetermined, logic suggests that to optimize the probability of favorable outcomes interventions should have the capacity to address the multiple risk factors contributing to the problem. For example, cardiovascular disease has multiple risk factors, including diet, exercise, stress, and substance use. Assuming that the goal is to minimize the probability of a heart attack, the optimal set of interventions would have the capacity to influence each of the pertinent risk factors.

Likewise, a broad consensus has been achieved among researchers regarding the variables that influence the development and maintenance of antisocial behavior in children and adolescents (Loeber & Farrington, 1998). These factors include individual youth characteristics (e.g., weak verbal skills, favorable attitudes toward antisocial behavior), family functioning (e.g., discipline, affect), caregiver functioning (e.g., mental health, substance abuse), peer relations (e.g., rejection, association with deviant peers), school performance, indigenous family supports, and neighborhood characteristics (e.g., criminal subculture). Hence, to optimize the probability of decreasing antisocial behavior, an intervention should have the capacity to address pertinent risk factors across the youth's social network (i.e., family, peers, school, support system).

Unfortunately, the vast majority of mental health interventions address only a limited subset of pertinent risk factors. For example, although cognitive-behavioral therapy is a well-respected evidence-based intervention, this approach addresses only a small subset of the determinants of serious antisocial behavior, and hence has little chance of being effective even when provided by highly skilled clinicians. The probability of success is even lower for interventions that do not address known risk factors (e.g., psychodynamic therapies) or interventions that exacerbate risks factors (e.g., placing antisocial youths together in groups; Arnold & Hughes, 1999; Dishion, McCord, & Poulin, 1999).

A key feature of MST is its capacity to address the multiple risk factors present in a particular case (hence the name "multisystemic"). Importantly, these risk factors are addressed in a highly individualized and strategic fashion. MST does not include "modules" of interventions aimed at particular systems such as the family and peers. Rather, as described in Chapter 2, MST requires a careful and ecologically based functional analysis of identified problems. Interventions are then selected strategically to provide maximum leverage for achieving a specified goal. Thus, the interventions are comprehensive, but individualized.

In addition, the development of protective factors is important to the maintenance of therapeutic change. In general, protective factors pertain to the emotional connections in the family, the family's connections with a strong indigenous social support network, and the development of youth educational and vocational skills and prosocial peer relations. MST attends explicitly to these protective factors as discussed in Chapters 2–4.

## MST Eliminates Barriers to Service Access and Treatment Generalization

Treatment can not be effective if it is not delivered. Youths with serious emotional and behavioral problems and their families have many legitimate reasons for not attending facility-based treatment services. Such families often have long histories of receiving ineffective services. Logistical problems with transportation, lack of flexibility in appointment times (e.g., few evening and weekend hours), and difficulty obtaining childcare often interfere with session attendance. Similarly, many families of children with serious emotional disturbance experience multiple stressors (e.g., poverty, housing difficulties, employment problems) that interfere with their capacity to attend scheduled meetings.

MST specifically aims to overcome barriers to service access as an important step toward first engaging the family in treatment and then achieving treatment goals. The home-based model of service delivery used by MST programs provides an excellent mechanism for delivering services with high ecological validity. Treatment is delivered where problems occur: in the home, at school, and in other community settings. Hence, rather than hoping that treatment gains will generalize from the office or residential placement to the home, MST therapists work directly to change those contexts that are contributing to identified problems. Therapists are available during evening and weekend hours, and MST programs provide crisis coverage 24 hours per day, 7 days per week. Therapists have low caseloads (four to six families per clinician), which allows them the time they need to engage with and provide intensive services for challenging families.

Importantly, the home-based model of service delivery also provides more valid information needed for treatment planning and evaluation. For example, interacting in a family's living room for 30 minutes arguably provides the therapist with more valid and useful assessment data than 10 hours of psychological testing with an individual youth. Valid assessment information increases the probability that effective interventions can be planned. Similarly, the home-based model of service delivery can provide more valid clinical outcome data. For example, talking about gains in child management practices with a parent in an office is a very different experience than observing such gains in the living room with the family present.

## MST Uses Evidence-Based Interventions

MST does not use a unique set of interventions. Rather, MST borrows from the best of the evidence-based treatments. As described recently by reviewers (Burns, Hoagwood, & Mrazek, 1999; DHHS, 1999; Weisz & Jensen, 1999), several intervention models have reasonable empirical support for decreasing the symptomatology and improving the functioning of children and adolescents with emotional and behavioral difficulties. These models include several variations of cognitive-behavioral therapy (CBT), behavior therapy, and selected pharmacological treatments.

MST uses these interventions, however, within a programmatic context and treatment philosophy that contrasts with the ways in which evidenced-based interventions are usually delivered. For example, programs that use evidenced-based treatments are rarely committed to overcoming barriers to service access. Similarly, most of these interventions are delivered within a relatively narrow conceptual framework. CBT, for example, is typically delivered to a child by a therapist in an office. Within the MST model, however, if a cognitive change is deemed a necessary step toward meeting ultimate treatment goals, the MST therapist would usually try to teach the caregiver to teach the youth the CBT strategies. Although the therapist is certainly better equipped to promote development of cognitive skills in the youth, teaching the caregiver to teach the youth helps to change the family's broader social ecology in ways that increase the likelihood of maintaining favorable outcomes. In addition, as described subsequently, MST programs view the caregiver as the key to achieving long-term outcomes, emphasize accountability of the provider for engaging families and achieving outcomes, and include intensive and ongoing quality assurance systems. These features are not characteristic of most evidence-based services as currently configured.

## MST Views the Caregiver as Key to Long-Term Outcomes

MST views the caregiver as the primary determinant of long-term clinical outcomes for referred children and adolescents. Hence, the majority of clinical resources are devoted to determining the barriers to effective parenting and to developing and implementing strategies to overcome these barriers. This perspective assumes, as is usually the case, that parenting has not been very effective if the youth is at imminent risk of out-of-home placement. Thus, within the MST model, clinicians determine the factors in the caregivers' lives that are interfering with their capacity to provide necessary nurturance, monitoring, and discipline for their child, as well as caregiver strengths that might be leveraged to enhance parenting competency. Examples of the former factors include parental substance abuse, untreated mental health disorders, physical limitations, high stress, low social support, and skill deficits. Examples of the latter factors include loving the child, the capacity to hold down a job, a supportive extended family, and social skills. Strengths are used to address barriers and facilitate the implementation of planned interventions.

Although viewing caregivers as critical to successful outcomes is central to family systems theories of behavior change and the philosophical bases of system of care reforms (Stroul & Friedman, 1996), mental health services for children have traditionally placed parents on the periphery of treatment or viewed caregivers as the problem, not the solution. Indeed, many mental health professionals (more than one of the present authors included) entered the field of child mental health because they truly enjoyed working with children and adolescents. Concomitantly, many of these professionals were not particularly fond of working with adults, especially adults who might have substance abuse problems or who might physically abuse their children. Hence, making the shift from the child as the primary client to the family as the client, as required by MST, can be extremely difficult for many professionals. This shift, however, reflects a fundamental tenet of MST. If therapeutic gains are to be maintained following treatment, the social ecology surrounding the child must be changed to support those gains. The child's caregivers are essential to this process.

## MST Assumes Accountability for Engaging Families and Achieving Clinical Outcomes

Currently, mental health providers have almost no accountability for engaging families in treatment or for youth outcomes. Difficult-to-engage families are considered "resistant," and their treatment may be terminated after several missed appointments. Similarly, clinicians rarely assume accountability for failing to achieve treatment goals. Rather, qualities of the child, family, or social environment are used to explain the lack of clinical progress.

Indeed, the lack of accountability of mental health providers has been institutionalized. Graduate programs rarely emphasize the teaching of evidence-based practices, and graduate degrees are largely certificates to practice as one desires until retirement. No performance criteria related to client outcomes need to be met to maintain clinical licenses. Professional guilds resist efforts to move to performance-based outcome criteria. Few other segments of the U.S. economy eschew accountability for outcomes with such effectiveness. Plumbers are held responsible for fixing leaks, the success rates of surgeons are tracked, and manufacturers track the quality of their products.

Increasing accountability of mental health providers is a vital step toward improving child and family outcomes. High accountability should be a feature of each MST program. Therapists, supervisors, and programs, however, can not be held accountable for outcomes unless they are provided with the tools, clinical support, and organizational structure they need to be successful. A lone practitioner can not be expected to effectively treat 20 children at imminent risk of placement and their families, and the many serious clinical challenges such families present. Hence, central features of MST programs include low caseloads, intensive training, well-specified supervision, and ongoing support from MST expert consultants. The issues of clinical support and quality assurance are discussed next.

## MST Implements a Strong Quality Assurance System

The vast majority of mental health services in the United States are delivered by bachelor's- and master's-level practitioners. Expecting any single clinician, master's level or otherwise, to possess the broad range of skills needed to treat the most difficult clinical cases in the nation is unrealistic. Children at imminent risk of placement and their families can present a broad range of extremely challenging problems, including substance dependence, extensive trauma histories, severe and persistent mental illnesses, relationship difficulties, social isolation, and significant cognitive and skill deficits.

To address the broad range of serious clinical problems that are seen by clinicians, MST programs provide intensive clinical support that is organized as a quality assurance system. Described more extensively in Chapter 9, the MST quality assurance system includes several interrelated components. The assessment and intervention process is manualized and focuses on a set of nine treatment principles that establish the playing field for therapist behaviors. Likewise, supervisory and consultation processes are manualized for the MST supervisors and expert MST consultants. Such manualization provides a clear framework for program implementation. In addition, extensive organizational consultation is provided to emerging MST programs to assure the provision of necessary resources (e.g., funding, low caseloads, interagency collaboration). On-site clinical supervisors are trained in the MST model of supervision, which focuses on child outcomes and treatment fidelity; and MST consultants facilitate the performance of supervisors on a weekly basis. Supervisors are responsible for the professional development of therapists (e.g., developing skills in marital therapy or CBT), and consultants are responsible for developing the supervisory skills of the supervisors. Moreover, the adherence of therapists and supervisors to MST protocols is monitored continuously through an Internet-based measurement system *mstinstitute.org*. Caregivers rate therapists on adherence to MST treatment principles, and therapists rate supervisors on fidelity to the MST supervisory protocol. Currently, as discussed in Chapter 9, MST programs are moving to a quality improvement system (see Bickman, 1999), in which fidelity and short-term outcomes are assessed continuously, and the resulting information is used to guide administrative decisions regarding staff performance and resource allocation.

### Summary

MST does not include any truly "unique" ideas. Rather, MST programs take advantage of the existing mental health knowledge base (e.g., child psychopathology literature, literature on evidence-based practices) and features of the corporate world that have improved product quality (e.g., performance accountability, quality improvement systems). Similarly, recognizing that barriers to service access must be overcome to deliver a treatment and that caregivers play pivotal roles in most children's lives are not profound insights. Traditionally, however, mental health has traveled down a very different set of paths. MST is attempting to develop and validate detailed and comprehensive maps showing the paths to youth and family outcomes.

## THE ROLE OF MST IN TREATING MENTAL HEALTH PROBLEMS

This section focuses on mental health problems that have not usually been emphasized in MST programs for serious juvenile offenders. Broadly, these difficulties come under the headings of "mood disorders" and "anxiety disorders." Historically, the mental health community has taken an individually oriented approach to treating these mental health problems. The literature, however, suggests that these problems are not solely determined by individual biology or cognitions. Rather, at least for the population of children and adolescents at risk of placement, these problems are intertwined with many of the same social-ecological variables that place highly antisocial youths at risk for placement.

## U.S. Surgeon General's Report and MST: Synonymous Underlying Assumptions

The U.S. Surgeon General's Report on Children and Mental Health (DHHS, 1999) concluded that several assumptions should guide our understanding and treatment of children's mental health and illness. First, "psychopathology in childhood arises from the complex, multi-layered interactions of specific characteristics of the child (including biological, psychological, and genetic factors), his or her environment (including parent, sibling, and family relations, peer and neighborhood factors, school and community factors, and the larger social–cultural context), and the specific manner in which these factors interact with and shape each other over the course of development" (p. 127). Hence, consistent with social-ecological theory (Bronfenbrenner, 1979) and MST conceptualizations of behavior, mental health problems are viewed as multi-determined and linked reciprocally with important features of the child's social ecology.

A second assumption is that children (and families) strive to adapt to the contexts in which they are embedded. Thus, when environments are chaotic or not supportive of healthy functioning, children's and families' adaptations may seem pathological. This assumption is a cornerstone of MST theory. As described more extensively in Chapter 2, MST practitioners strive to understand how identified problems "fit," or make sense, in the child's and the family's ecological context. The development of such understanding is an essential step toward the design of effective interventions.

A third assumption from the Surgeon General's Report (DHHS, 1999) pertains to the critical importance of the child's caregiving environment. Parents or other caregivers play vital roles in the short- and long-term development of healthy socioemotional functioning. This assumption supports the emphasis that MST places on viewing caregivers as the key to short- and long-term child functioning.

Importantly, the Surgeon General's Report (DHHS, 1999) drew out the treatment implications of these assumptions. Such implications essentially describe the clinical foci of MST. That is, interventions must move beyond static and simplistic diagnostic terms to address the complex array of interrelated factors in the youth and across his or her social ecology that are related to the onset, maintenance, or amelioration of mental health problems. The following sections briefly describe the pertinence of a social-ecological view of child mental health problems that have traditionally been treated from an individual emphasis.

## Social-Ecological Nature of Mental Health Problems

The multidetermined nature of externalizing problems such as conduct disorder, delinquency, and substance abuse has been explicated by decades of correlational, longitudinal, and experimental research, with reviewers (e.g., Loeber & Farrington, 1998) drawing consistent conclusions regarding the key predictors of antisocial behavior and the implications of these predictors for treatment. To a large extent, MST interventions for antisocial behavior (Henggeler et al., 1998) are based on this literature.

The literature on the determinants of mental health problems such as depression and anxiety, however, is much less extensive. Although a relatively greater proportion of variance in antisocial behavior might be explained by contextual variables and a relatively greater proportion of the variance of internalizing problems might be explained by biological and cognitive variables, the expression of biological predispositions is influenced by context (e.g., caregiver functioning, stress), and that context often contributes independently to the development of mental health difficulties (DHHS, 1999).

## DEPRESSION

Major reviews (Birmaher, Ryan, Williamson, Brent, & Kaufman, 1996; Birmaher, Ryan, Williamson, Brent, Kaufman, Dahl, et al., 1996) of research on childhood and adolescent depression (major depressive disorder and dysthymic disorder) have concluded that the onset, duration, and recurrence of childhood depression are associated with genetic loadings, youth cognitive style (e.g., negative attributions, pessimistic attitudinal style), caregiver problems (e.g., parental psychopathology), family relations (e.g., conflict, rejection, low positive affect), and stressful life events in the context of low social support. As noted earlier, treatments of childhood and adolescent depression have traditionally focused on the level of the individual child. Here, CBT has relatively strong empirical support for effectiveness (Reinecke, Ryan, & DuBois, 1998), and selective serotonin reuptake inhibitors (SSRIs; see Chapter 6) have shown considerable promise (Burns et al., 1999; DHHS, 1999; Weisz & Jensen, 1999). Nevertheless, the aforementioned reviewers have concluded that multifaceted interventions are needed to address the high degree of comorbidity and negative psychosocial and academic consequences of childhood depression as well as the mental health problems of the youths' caregivers.

## BIPOLAR DISORDER

Bipolar disorder is associated with serious emotional regulation problems; psychosocial difficulties across the youth's family, peer, school, and neighborhood contexts; and psychiatric comorbidities such as substance abuse, anxiety disorders, and conduct disorders (American Academy of Child and Adolescent Psychiatry [AACAP], 1997). The AACAP treatment guidelines, therefore, emphasize the importance of multimodal treatment integrating medications with interventions aimed at the multiple psychosocial difficulties. Unfortunately, virtually no research has been conducted on psychosocial treatments of youths with bipolar disorder, and research on pharmacological treatment is scarce. Although lithium has some support for use with children and adolescents, serious safety concerns are evident when prescribed for youth in families that have difficulty monitoring dosage and attending appointments (Burns et al., 1999). The serious and challenging problems presented by children and adolescents with bipolar disorder in conjunction with scant knowledge regarding effective treatments suggest that intensive, comprehensive, and well-conceived interventions are needed for such youths and their families.

## ANXIETY

Research on the development and treatment of anxiety disorders (e.g., generalized anxiety disorder, social phobia, separation anxiety disorder) in children and adolescents is not as well developed as in other areas of mental health services (Burns et al., 1999; Ollendick & King, 1998; DHHS, 1999; Weisz & Jensen, 1999). Reviewers have concluded, however, that Kendall's individually oriented CBT for childhood anxiety (e.g., Kendall et al., 1997) shows considerable promise. Moreover, recent research has affirmed the role of families (especially caregivers) in maintaining children's anxieties through negative feedback and restriction (Ollendick & King, 1998). Training parents in specific skills to help manage their child's anxieties has significantly enhanced the outcomes of Kendall's CBT program (Barrett, Dadds, & Rapee, 1996). These findings support the importance of context and caregivers in treating mental health problems.

## OBSESSIVE–COMPULSIVE DISORDER

Also classified as an anxiety disorder, obsessive–compulsive disorder (OCD) is a quintessential neuropsychiatric disorder (March & Leonard, 1996), as supported from genetic, neuroimaging, and neurotransmitter and neuroendocrine studies. Consistent with this perspective, SSRIs have proven effective in treating children and adolescents with OCD (Burns et al., 1999; DHHS, 1999; Weisz & Jensen, 1999), and cognitive behavior therapy is considered a useful component of treatment. March and Leonard (1996) noted that OCD can severely disrupt social and academic functioning, and that much work remains to be done in transferring the effective treatment technologies from research to community practice.

## POSTTRAUMATIC STRESS DISORDER

Posttraumatic stress disorder (PTSD) is an increasing concern for clinicians working in communities with high rates of violence and victimization (Pfefferbaum, 1997). Exposure to trauma, however, does not necessarily lead to symptoms, and several factors (e.g., severity of trauma, emotional and physical proximity to trauma, parental response) seem to mediate the association between trauma exposure and symptoms. In addition, children with PTSD often have comorbid problems, such as conduct disorder and anxiety disorders. Although many types of interventions have been used to treat PTSD, empirical support is evident solely for variations of CBT (AACAP, 1998). Specifically, CBT interventions that provide exposure to the trauma through direct discussion, desensitization, and cognitive reframing have been effective. Moreover, because caregiver reactions (e.g., support vs. distress) are important predictors of children's response to trauma, the inclusion of caregivers in treatment is deemed important in symptom resolution (AACAP, 1998).

## ATTENTION-DEFICIT/HYPERACTIVITY DISORDER

The knowledge base on attention-deficit/hyperactivity disorder (ADHD) is extensive and reviewers have drawn consistent conclusions (Burns et al., 1999; DHHS, 1999; Weisz & Jensen, 1999). Children with ADHD often have psychiatric comorbidity and experience a myriad of difficulties across home, peer, and school settings. Psychostimulants have proven highly effective at decreasing the core symptoms of ADHD. Intensive behavioral interventions (but not CBT) in family and school settings have produced modest improvements in core ADHD symptoms and in problems associated with ADHD (e.g., oppositional behavior, parent–child relations, internalizing symptoms). In consideration of the results of the NIMH Multimodal Treatment Study (Jensen, 2001; Multimodal Treatment Study of Children with ADHD Cooperative Group, 1999), medication alone was the most efficient and cost-effective intervention for youths with ADHD and few concomitant problems. On the other hand, for children and adolescents with ADHD and co-occurring emotional or behavioral difficulties, medication in combination with contingency-oriented behavioral therapy involving caregivers and teachers was more effective.

## When Is MST Indicated?

MST is most appropriate for children and adolescents who are presenting complex, multifaceted, and challenging mental health and behavioral problems, especially problems that are costly to service systems. For example, MST has been traditionally applied to youths presenting serious antisocial behavior (e.g., violent offending, substance abuse) who were at high or imminent risk of out-of-home placements. Although these youths often had psychiatric comorbidities, the focus of treatment was on attenuating the serious antisocial behavior that was directly leading to the placement risk. Mental health problems were not ignored, but they were not usually the primary focus of treatment. Hence, psychiatry has played an important adjunctive, but not a primary, role in MST programs for serious juvenile offenders.

As MST developers and researchers adapted the model to treat youths presenting psychiatric emergencies (Henggeler, Rowland, et al., 1997, 1999; Rowland et al., 2000), the emphasis of MST interventions shifted to serious emotional problems, such as major depression and bipolar disorder, that were contributing substantially to the presenting psychiatric crisis (e.g., suicidal attempt). Hence, the primary focus for this population is on ameliorating the serious emotional disturbance. Because many youths with serious emotional disturbance also present serious antisocial behavior, behavior problems are often addressed, but not in every case. In treating youths with serious emotional disturbance, the role of psychiatry is at least substantive, and is often primary (see Chapters 5–7).

In regard to treating mental health problems, MST is indicated for youths presenting mental health difficulties that are sufficiently complex as to require relatively costly services in the short or long term. For example, an adolescent with major depression, a chaotic family structure, and impaired school functioning would probably be appropriate for MST. Likewise, a youth with an anxiety disorder and comorbidity for a significant externalizing disorder might be appropriate for MST. A youth with bipolar disorder, no comorbidities, and a chaotic family structure might be appropriate for MST in light of the importance of following medication protocols. Although MST inclusion criteria can not be exactly delineated, the rule of thumb is that MST services are intended for youth (and their families) presenting difficult and multifaceted problems that are not likely amenable to effective treatment from existing services and for which alternative institution-based services are costly.

## When Is MST Not Indicated?

MST is not indicated in cases where the sole use of other evidence-based treatments is sufficient. For example, an adolescent with OCD, no psychiatric comorbidities, and a supportive family does not need MST. An appropriate medication protocol and CBT should be sufficient to ameliorate the symptoms. Similarly, a child with ADHD, no significant comorbidities, and a supportive family would likely benefit most cost-effectively from appropriate medication. As another example, clinically effective and cost-effective intervention models (e.g., Webster-Stratton, 1998; Webster-Stratton & Hammond, 1997) are available for young children presenting disruptive behavior and their families.

MST is also not appropriate for delivery in institutional settings such as inpatient psychiatric units and residential treatment centers. A central tenet of MST pertains to the importance of helping caregivers restructure the natural ecologies of children and adolescents to support constructive and responsible behavior. Natural ecologies, such as homes, schools, neighborhoods, and social support systems can not be addressed with any validity from the confines of an institution. Learning how to adapt to an institutional placement has little generalization to real-world settings. MST would be appropriate, however, as the aftercare for an early release from the institution.

## CONCLUSION

The success of MST in treating serious antisocial behavior provides valuable lessons that are applicable to the field of mental health services for children. Specifically, services should address known risk and protective factors, overcome barriers to treatment access, endeavor to empower caregivers, use evidence-based interventions, assume accountability for outcomes, and incorporate strong quality assurance systems to promote treatment fidelity. Such emphases are fully consistent with the directions advocated by leading reviewers and policymakers in the field of mental health services. More importantly, the validity of these emphases is supported by emerging evidence of the effectiveness of MST in treating serious emotional disturbance in children and adolescents, as described in Chapter 8.

# CHAPTER 2

# MST Principles and Process

Children with serious emotional disturbance and their families often present a multitude of interrelated problems. This chapter describes the criteria that MST therapists use to prioritize treatment goals, design interventions to meet those goals, and evaluate the success of those interventions. These criteria are operationalized in protocols that are flexible yet include significant structure and outcome monitoring to enhance therapist and family capacity to achieve treatment goals.

With each new referral to an MST program, the MST therapist has the opportunity of a lifetime: the lifetime of a youth and his or her family. An effective MST therapist helps a family to change the course of a child's life. The privileges, responsibilities, and challenges inherent in doing so are urgent and awesome. Urgent, because the youth in question is typically headed toward a life course of multiple disruptive out-of-home placements, educational and vocational failure, interpersonal problems, and deterioration in mental and physical health. Awesome because so little of what is available to youth and families in most communities can effectively alter that life course, and because many attempts made by the youth, his or her family, school, and mental health providers have already failed. The privileges and challenges presented with each new referral also vary in accordance with the particular strengths and needs of each youth, his or her family, and the family's context. Accordingly, the intervention strategies and techniques implemented by the MST therapist, family members, relatives, friends, or school personnel are individualized to the youth and his or her context.

The individualization of MST occurs within the parameters provided by nine treatment principles and a systematic and ongoing assessment and treatment process. That process brings the scientific method of hypothesis testing to the complexities of each referral. Referred to as the *Analytic Process* (a.k.a. the "Do-Loop"; see Figure 2.1), this method encourages clinicians to generate specific hypotheses about what combination of factors sustains a particular problem behavior, provide evidence to support the hypotheses, test the hypotheses by intervening, collect

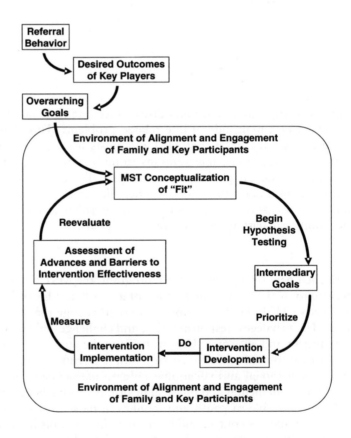

**FIGURE 2.1.** MST analytic process (a.k.a. Do-Loop).

data to assess the impact of the intervention, and use that data to begin the assessment process again. The sources of information from which hypotheses are drawn include: the knowledge base on the individual, family, peer, school, and neighborhood factors that contribute to serious clinical problems; and reports by the youth, family members, and key members of the social context and the therapist's observations of all these. Hypotheses are also informed by social-ecological and systems theories of human behavior. This chapter describes the MST treatment principles and analytic process, the advantages of delivering MST through a home-based model of service delivery, and the quality assurance processes designed to support the effective implementation of MST by providers in community-based sites.

## MST TREATMENT PRINCIPLES

*Treatment specification* is the process used to translate ideas about what causes clinical problems into actions designed to solve or more effectively manage these problems. For treatments that have been validated in scientific studies, ideas about what causes problems are derived from well-established research findings and a theoretical framework that is consistent with those findings. As described in Chapter 1, the social-ecological framework that informs MST is consistent with decades of research demonstrating the multiple predictors of serious behavior problems in youth. Treatment specification identifies core intervention procedures to solve or manage those problems and the expected outcomes of those procedures.

Compared to other children's mental health services (e.g., intensive case management, other models of home-based services, "wraparound" services, residential treatment, and psychiatric hospitalization), MST is very well specified. Relative to psychotherapy models that focus primarily on one factor contributing to a behavior problem with specific and sequential intervention steps, MST is relatively loosely specified. In contrast with therapy approaches such as parent–child management or social problem-solving skills training, for example, step-by-step or session-by-session guides are not used to implement MST.

To address the needs of youths and families with multiple complex problems, the MST therapist must individualize strategies to capitalize on the strengths and limitations of the youth, his or her family, and the surrounding context. Consequently, the combination of intervention techniques applied, and the expected impact of intervention procedures, varies in accordance with the circumstances of each youth and family. Thus, to fully specify all procedures used in MST to address a broad

## TABLE 2.1. MST Treatment Principles

*Principle 1*: The primary purpose of assessment is to understand the "fit" between the identified problems and their broader systemic context.

*Principle 2*: Therapeutic contacts should emphasize the positive and should use systemic strengths as levers for change.

*Principle 3*: Interventions should be designed to promote responsible behavior and decrease irresponsible behavior among family members.

*Principle 4*: Interventions should be present-focused and action-oriented, targeting specific and well-defined problems.

*Principle 5*: Interventions should target sequences of behavior within and between multiple systems that maintain the identified problems.

*Principle 6:* Interventions should be developmentally appropriate and fit the developmental needs of the youth.

*Principle 7*: Interventions should be designed to require daily or weekly effort by family members.

*Principle 8*: Intervention efficacy is evaluated continuously from multiple perspectives with providers assuming accountability for overcoming barriers to successful outcomes.

*Principle 9*: Interventions should be designed to promote treatment generalization and long-term maintenance of therapeutic change by empowering caregivers to address family members' needs across multiple systemic contexts.

range of youth, family, and contextual problems would be an unproductive way to delineate the treatment model. Such detailed specification would not allow the therapist and treatment team the flexibility they need to address a complex array of problems effectively.

To balance adequate specification of the model with responsiveness to the needs and strengths of each youth and family, principles are used to guide the MST assessment and intervention process (see Table 2.1). By virtue of the flexibility inherent in these principles, MST therapists—most of whom are seasoned professionals before joining an MST team—have the freedom to use their strengths in the service of the family. By virtue of their brevity (all nine principles fit on two sides of a business card), the principles can be readily referenced by therapists during clinical supervision and in the field. Moreover, therapist adherence to these principles can be readily assessed through caregiver reports (discussed in the quality assurance section of this chapter).

The first two MST principles focus assessment and intervention efforts on the multiple factors within the youth's ecology that can help make sense of why problems are occurring (Principle 1) and on identifying strengths of the youth, family, and surrounding context that can be used to promote change (Principle 2). Principle 3 highlights the importance of interventions that increase responsible behavior. Principles 4 and 5 emphasize the clear and objective definition of problems targeted for change and the use of present-focused and action-oriented approaches to changing interactions that sustain these problems. Principle 6 draws attention to the developmental aspects of individualization of treatment. Principle 7 emphasizes the centrality of daily effort to change. The last two principles focus on the need for continuous evaluation of, and provider accountability for, the impact of interventions, and for the implementation of interventions that will be sustainable after treatment ends.

Importantly, the MST principles are consistent with key aspects of empirically based treatment approaches for youth and families (e.g., strategic, structural, and behavioral family systems approaches; behavioral parent training; cognitive-behavioral therapies). The principles embody the problem-focused, present-focused, and action-oriented emphases of behavioral and cognitive-behavioral treatment techniques; the contextual emphases of pragmatic family systems therapies; and the importance of client–clinician collaboration and treatment generalization emphasized in system of care and consumer philosophies. In MST, however, these evidence-based interventions, which have historically focused on a limited aspect of the youth's social ecology (e.g., the cognitions or problem-solving skills of the individual youth; the discipline strategies of a parent; family interactions, but not interactions between the family and other systems), are integrated into a social-ecological framework. Moreover, MST interventions are delivered where the problems and their potential solutions are found: at home, at school, and in the neighborhood rather than in a therapist's office.

MST interventions are tailored to the specific strengths and weaknesses of each youth's family, peer, school, and community contexts. In addition, and as described in subsequent chapters, biological contributors to identified problems are identified and psychopharmacological treatment is integrated with psychosocial treatment. In contrast to "combined" (e.g., Kazdin, 1996; Kazdin, Siegel, & Bass, 1992) and multicomponent approaches to treatment (e.g., Liddle, 1996), however, MST interventions are not delivered as separate elements or self-contained modules. Rather, throughout the 3–5 months of MST treatment, interventions are strategically selected and integrated in ways hypothesized to maximize their synergistic interaction. For example, parents with permissive parenting practices often need instrumental and emotional support from spouses, kin, and/or friends to change their parenting practices in the face of significant protests from the youth. Thus, therapist and parent might work together to mend fences between the parent and an estranged relative before trying to implement new rules and consequences for a youth, so that the relative can actively support the parent when she first tries to implement new rules and consequences.

### From Principles to Practice: A Brief Introduction

Subsequent chapters describe the application of MST principles to the treatment of youths with serious emotional disturbances and their families. The purpose of the following description of Jennifer is to provide a sampling of how the MST treatment principles are applied.

Jennifer Stone was a 15-year-old white female referred to the MST program jointly by the local child protection and juvenile justice agencies after domestic violence and incorrigibility charges were filed against her. The domestic violence charge stemmed from a fight in which Jennifer broke her 13-year-old half-sister's wrist and tried to hit her stepmother, Mary, with a pan when she tried to intervene. The incorrigibility charges stemmed from several runaway incidents also reported to authorities by Mary. Jennifer was frequently truant from school and had been suspended repeatedly for fighting with peers. During the previous school year, Jennifer had been hospitalized for a psychiatric evaluation following a school incident in which she physically threatened a teacher. At that time, Jennifer was diagnosed with depression and ADHD. Jennifer lived with her father, John, her stepmother, Mary, and her three half-siblings: Anna (13), Jacob (6), and Kate (3). John had obtained sole custody of Jennifer when she was 12; at that time, Jennifer's mother, Brenda, entered a court-ordered drug rehabilitation program. Following her release from that program, Brenda continued to have substance abuse problems that interfered with her ability to retain employment and stable housing. Brenda intermittently visited her daughter. Mary had a congenital heart problem that required frequent medical attention and compromised her physical stamina.

### PRINCIPLE 1: FINDING THE FIT

Consistent with social-ecological theory and research on the multiple determinants of serious problems in youth, a fundamental premise of MST is that behavior makes sense in its context. Thus, the primary purpose of the ongoing MST assessment process is to understand the "fit" between the identified problems and their broader systemic context. For each youth referred to MST, the therapist attempts to determine the specific combination of factors that sustain identified problems and thus can be used to help attenuate them.

As described in the MST analytic process section of this chapter, interview and observational methods are used to identify this combination of factors. The therapist interviews family members, relatives, neighbors, and friends in the family's social network, teachers and other school personnel (e.g., coaches, principals, lunch room attendants), and individuals involved in community activities attended by the youth and family (e.g., church, mosque, or synagogue; recreation center). The therapist observes interactions among family members and those involving the youth and pertinent family members in school and community settings.

In Jennifer's case, the therapist interviewed Jennifer's father, step-mother, mother, grandmother, and teachers, and observed interactions involving Jennifer in the home and at school. She also observed interactions between the adults in Jennifer's life when Jennifer was not present. These interviews and observations, which occurred within the first 2–3 days after Jennifer was referred for treatment, led the therapist to identify several factors associated with Jennifer's physical violence at home and school.

A graphic depiction of these fit factors appears in Figure 2.2. First, information from Jennifer's parents, grandmother, and teachers indicated that Jennifer had always had considerable difficulties sustaining attention and controlling impulses at school and at home. This information led the team to tentatively support the hypothesis that *ADHD* was a contributing factor. Furthermore, all observers confirmed that Jennifer did not take her medication (Ritalin). Information about possible depression was mixed, with Jennifer denying feelings of sadness, and parents and teachers reporting irritability and occasional behaviors (acting "spacey," slowed speech, inappropriate laughter) that might signal substance use rather than depression. Thus, second, the therapist added *"possible substance use"* to the list of contributing factors, and suspended opinion about the depression pending further observation and consultation with the psychiatrist working with the team. Third, Jennifer had begun to hang out with a couple of *"tough girls"* about a year after she moved in permanently with her father; one of the girls was well known for picking fights, stealing, and dating a known drug dealer. These girls also harbored Jennifer when she ran away from home. Fourth, Jennifer had nearly unlimited access to these peers because her father and stepmother rarely monitored her whereabouts. The *lack of monitoring*, in turn, was a product of long work hours and a permissive parenting style for John, lack of stamina and the demands associated with caring for the other children for Mary, and the conflicting parenting styles of John and Mary, who was more authoritative than John in

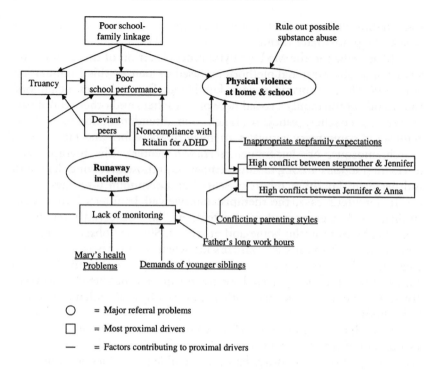

FIGURE 2.2. Initial conceptualization of "fit" for Jennifer.

her parenting practices. Fifth, *verbal conflict* in the family was high, particularly between Jennifer and Mary and between Jennifer and Anna.
Other fit factors included *poor school performance*, which, in turn, was
directly linked with Jennifer's ADHD, and indirectly linked with the truancy and aggression that resulted in repeated suspensions. The relationship between school personnel and family members was tense, at best:
Jennifer's reputation among teachers was poor, and the teachers experienced John as inaccessible and Mary as unable to change Jennifer's
behavior.

## PRINCIPLE 2: STRENGTHS AS LEVERS FOR CHANGE

Although families of children with serious problems are faced with many
challenges, they also possess many strengths. The former cannot be successfully addressed without harnessing the latter. Few individuals in any
walk of life are eager to engage in relationships built primarily around
the identification of their weaknesses. Unfortunately, mental health and

social service professionals and agencies often focus on deficits rather than strengths, thereby failing to engage families in the treatment process. MST therapist contacts with the youth, his or her family, and other key individuals in their ecology emphasize the positive, and therapeutic interventions use systemic and individual strengths as levers for change. Maintaining a strength-focused approach in the midst of complex and challenging situations requires that the entire team (e.g., other therapists, supervisor) share this strength-focused perspective.

Jennifer and her family possessed several strengths. At the *family* level, John loved his daughter, and Mary was concerned about Jennifer's well-being, though her concern about her own safety and that of her children sometimes superseded the concern about Jennifer. Although strained by the demands of work, children, Mary's health problem, and conflict about parenting styles, the marriage was relatively strong and long-standing (13 years). In addition, although Mary didn't have the affective bond needed to parent Jennifer effectively, her authoritative parenting style offered a credible model for John, who was permissive. Jennifer's maternal grandmother, with whom Jennifer had sometimes lived when her mother's housing was unstable, was willing to be helpful as long as Jennifer did not come to live with her again. At *school*, the school-based mental health counselor had a soft spot for Jennifer, and was willing to work with the MST therapist and teachers to develop alternatives to suspension for some of the behaviors that were inappropriate and irritating but not violent. With respect to *peers*, Jennifer had demonstrated some interest in electric guitar and studio music before hooking up with the tough crowd, and she occasionally contacted one relatively prosocial acquaintance that lived in her maternal grandmother's neighborhood. Thus, despite significant and challenging problems, Jennifer, her family, and their social context contained several significant strengths that could be used to facilitate change.

## PRINCIPLE 3: INCREASING RESPONSIBLE BEHAVIOR

As with all serious or chronic health conditions, psychiatric, behavioral, and emotional problems can be managed more or less effectively. Effective management of such problems requires the youth and others in the social ecology to exercise additional responsibilities. MST therapists assist caregivers and other key players to help the youth behave responsibly, even when faced with limitations imposed by a psychiatric illness. As illustrated in Jennifer's case, effective management of such limitations is a shared responsibility of the youth, his or her family, and others in their environment. For example, to effectively manage Jennifer's symptoms of ADHD, medication adherence is required. Jennifer should be attending school, performing to the best of her ability there, and handling the frustrations that might be associated with her ADHD. She should not be associating with friends who help get her into trouble. The father, stepmother, and school personnel should be responsible for facilitating medication management, sustaining school attendance, and monitoring Jennifer's peer connections. The responsibility to serve as primary parental authority, which resided with Mary for the children born to John and Mary, should be redirected to John when it comes to parenting Jennifer (because Mary and Jennifer had not established the affective bond needed for effective parenting). John and Mary, on the other hand, should share the responsibility for managing half-sibling conflict. Framed from the perspective of increasing such responsible behavior, none of these treatment goals seemed unrealistic.

## PRINCIPLE 4: PRESENT FOCUSED, ACTION ORIENTED, WELL DEFINED

MST interventions are designed to change the everyday transactions and circumstances that sustain identified problems. The focus of each intervention should be clear and unambiguous. The intervention itself should be well specified, and whether the intervention achieves the desired effect should be equally clear—that is, observable. This present-focused action orientation contrasts with approaches that are primarily insight-oriented, past-focused, and of unlimited treatment length. Thus, although some of Jennifer's problem behaviors—such as impulsive behavior, physical aggression, irritability, and truancy—predated Jennifer's moving in with John and Mary, the therapist spent very little time talking about what life was like when Jennifer lived with her mother or grandmother. Instead, the therapist focused on the everyday events that enabled Jennifer to avoid taking medication for ADHD, engage in physical conflicts at home and at school, and stay connected with deviant peers. Intervention strategies focused initially on increasing the safety of family members by reducing family conflict, shifting parental authority for Jennifer from Mary to John, and increasing monitoring so that Jennifer would have less access to deviant peers and find it impossible to stay with them when she ran away from home.

## PRINCIPLE 5: TARGETING SEQUENCES OF BEHAVIOR

MST interventions target repeated sequences of interactions within the family, school, peer group, neighborhood, and community that maintain the identified problems. Equally importantly, interventions target problematic interactions between these systems. In this family, the interaction patterns immediately targeted for change were the conflicts between Jennifer and Anna and between Jennifer and Mary. These conflicts were related to one another. Common factors contributing to both were the inappropriate expectations both John and Mary held about blended families and their conflicting (permissive, authoritative) parenting styles. Therapy sessions and homework were directed toward establishing appropriate stepfamily expectations, resolving parenting inconsistencies, establishing John's role as the primary parental authority for Jennifer, and increasing positive affect between Mary and Jennifer. The conflict sequences also precipitated runaway incidents, but the willingness of peers and their parents to harbor Jennifer when she ran away extended the relevant sequences of behavior outside the family system. Thus, interventions were designed to help John and Mary work with these parents to prevent harboring.

## PRINCIPLE 6: DEVELOPMENTALLY APPROPRIATE

Children and their caregivers have different needs at different times in their lives. Thus, MST intervention strategies are tailored to the physical, intellectual, social, and emotional needs of the children and their caregivers. For example, behavioral contingencies developed for 10-year-olds are different from those developed for 15-year-olds, new household rules may need to be posted in symbols rather than in words for a caregiver with a developmental disability. For Jennifer, age 15, such privileges as telephone time, taking the subway to see a friend in her grandmother's neighborhood, and earning money to buy items she valued were among contingencies developed by the therapist and parents to support medication compliance, school attendance and performance, and nonviolent responses to interpersonal problems. That is, when Jennifer took her medication as prescribed, attended school, and asked for schoolwork help from teachers and peers (all increases in responsible behavior on her part), the freedoms allowed her were in keeping with those afforded responsible age-mates.

## PRINCIPLE 7: CONTINUOUS EFFORT

Given the assumptions subsumed in the other principles—namely, that everyday interactions and circumstances maintain and can help attenuate identified problems—then anything less than everyday effort is likely to slow treatment progress. Thus, MST interventions are designed to require everyone involved in the daily life of a youth to work together diligently—weekly, if not daily—to achieve agreed-upon outcomes. Designing interventions that require such frequent effort also enables

therapists and family members to quickly detect and alter ineffective interventions and assess progress toward treatment goals. In Jennifer's
case, for example, compliance with ADHD medication was seen as critical to treatment success. Thus, a system of monitoring, rewards, and
consequences that required daily checking was established. Efforts to
shift some of the parenting responsibilities from Mary to John required
daily practice, initially in the presence of the therapist, and daily tracking of his efforts to enforce rules and to provide appropriate rewards
and consequences.

## PRINCIPLE 8: EVALUATION AND ACCOUNTABILITY

The effects of MST interventions are evaluated from multiple perspectives throughout the treatment process. The purpose of this principle is
to ensure that treatment progress and outcomes are objectively defined
and closely monitored, and that MST providers take responsibility for
identifying and overcoming barriers to treatment success. To assess
treatment progress (or lack thereof) in Jennifer's case, John obtained information on Jennifer's attendance and behavior (including fighting)
through daily checklist-type reports completed by teachers. The therapist obtained information on medication compliance, violent behavior,
and peer activities from Mary, John, grandmother, and the probation
and child protection workers assigned to the case. When progress was
elusive, the team undertook the responsibility of identifying and overcoming barriers to change (see next section).

## PRINCIPLE 9: GENERALIZATION

MST interventions are designed to promote the ability of individuals and
systems in the youth's natural ecology to sustain treatment gains. Although a variety of individuals in the social ecology (e.g., peers, teachers,
relatives, neighbors) affect a youth's well-being, the youth's caregivers
are the executive officers of the social ecology. Thus, MST interventions
are designed to empower caregivers to deal effectively with the inevitable
challenges of raising children. To this end, interventions accentuate the
strengths of caregivers, the youth, and other family members and build
the capacity of the caregivers and naturally occurring social supports to
effectively manage current and future problems.

For example, once John and Mary agreed to shift parenting roles,
the therapist and family included the grandmother and Mary's sister
(who lived in another city, but could be accessed by phone) in interventions that shifted parental authority from Mary to John. The purpose of
extended family involvement was to support John when he began taking

the lead and to support Mary in backing off. The medication and school monitoring plans were also shared with the grandmother, who agreed to let Jennifer come to her home if she and Anna or she and Mary began to inch toward conflict before John came home from work. The therapist moved out of the school–home communications circle within the first 3 weeks of treatment, and instead coached John and Mary to work with the school mental health counselor and principal, both of whom would continue to work at the school long after MST ended.

## MST ANALYTIC PROCESS

The MST treatment process entails interrelated steps that connect the ongoing assessment of the fit of identified problems with the development and implementation of interventions. The steps in this process are depicted in Figure 2.1, known as the "MST Do-Loop." Prior to supervision each week, clinicians summarize each case on a Weekly Progress Summary, which is organized in terms of the steps on the Do-Loop. Thus, therapists report on:

- Reasons for referral.
- Desired outcomes and overarching/primary goals of treatment.
- The fit of identified problems.
- The intermediary goals (i.e., goals that represent steps toward achieving the overarching goals).
- Interventions developed and how they were implemented.
- Barriers to meeting the intermediary goals.
- Fit of advances and barriers (i.e., factors that contribute to successful achievement of the goal, factors that contribute to identified barriers to goal attainment).
- New intermediary goals for the upcoming weeks that build upon treatment advances and address observed barriers to treatment progress.

Hypothesis testing occurs throughout this process, beginning with the initial conceptualization of the fit of referral problems.

### Clarifying Reasons for Referral

As depicted in Figure 2.1, the ongoing MST assessment and intervention process begins with a clear understanding of the reasons for referral. To gain that understanding, MST therapists meet with family members and other key figures in the ecology (e.g., probation officers, teachers, etc.) to identify the problem behaviors that led to the referral. Common examples of problems identified include suicide threats; depressed and irritable behavior at school and at home; explosive physical outbursts that disrupt classroom, peer, or family functioning; fighting with peers; poor school performance; truancy and defiance toward teachers; substance abuse; and running away.

## Developing Overarching Goals

An overarching goal is an ultimate aim of treatment that:

- Eliminates or greatly reduces the frequency and intensity of a referral behavior (see above).
- Incorporates the desired outcomes of key participants (e.g., primary and secondary caregiver, teacher or principal, probation officer, judge, etc.).
- Can be measured directly.
- Is specified so that any outside observer would interpret the goal the same way and could determine whether the goal was met.

To establish such goals, clinicians should be able to pull from the desired outcomes of each key participant (caregiver, referral agencies, teachers, etc.) the common threads of an overarching goal. In the case of Jennifer, for example, the father, stepmother, and child welfare agency wanted physical fights at home to end, while school personnel focused on ending physical fights at school. Thus, an initial overarching goal was, "Stop physical fights at home and at school." Overarching goals often need to be prioritized. When a referred youth is both at imminent risk of harm to self and truant from school, ensuring safety from harm would be seen as more critical than ensuring regular school attendance in the early days of therapist involvement with the family. Overarching goals may be added or eliminated in accordance with information obtained as the clinician and family continue the assessment process. In the case of Jennifer, the sequences of interaction that supported fighting differed at home and at school, thus requiring separation of the original single goal into two goals that were met with different interventions.

## Fit of Identified Problems

Next, therapists develop a preliminary multisystemic explication of the fit of identified problems that encompasses the strengths and the weaknesses observed in each of the systems in the youth's ecology. Known as a "fit analysis," this process is depicted using a visual tool known as a

"fit circle." A specific behavior problem or interaction pattern is identified in the center of the circle, with arrows from possible contributing
factors pointing toward the circle. As Figure 2.2 shows, some factors
may contribute to more than one problem. The fit analysis becomes
more detailed as the clinician gathers information and makes observations about interactions within and between each system that directly
and indirectly influence identified problems. A common combination of
contributing factors to referral problems of youth with serious emotional disturbance (e.g., threatening harm to self or others, aggressive
behavior at home or school, running away) includes chronic parent–
child conflict; inconsistent parental discipline practices; poor parental
monitoring due to parental employment demands, substance abuse,
mental health problems, or lack of skill; peer reinforcement of irresponsible behavior; negative interactions between school personnel and family members; cognitive attribution biases of the youth; and biological
contributors such as ADHD. A sampling of strengths includes parental
concern about the youth's difficulties; strong emotional bond between
parent and child; parental employment; youth's interest in prosocial activities; youth's ability to get along with classmates who do well in
school; willingness of school personnel to work with a child or parent;
and relatives or friends willing to support parental efforts to manage the
youth's problems.

In Jennifer's case, for example, a fit circle would be developed for
each of the proximal drivers identified in Figure 2.2. Thus, "lack of
monitoring" would become the center of a fit circle, with Mary's health
problems, demands of younger siblings, father's long work hours, and
conflicting parenting styles identified initially as contributing factors.
Similarly, a separate fit circle would be developed to identify the factors
that contribute to "conflicting parenting styles" before interventions to
reduce conflict are designed.

### Hypothesis Development and Testing

Throughout the ongoing MST assessment and intervention process,
clinicians are encouraged to apply the scientific process of hypothesis development and testing. *Hypotheses* are hunches or theories that can be
expressed in terms that are concrete and measurable. Hypotheses are
initially developed on the basis of therapist observations of interaction
patterns and interviews with key participants in the youth's ecology. As
indicated in Figure 2.1, hypothesis development and testing begins at the
moment a clinician or family member uses a piece of information or an
observation to generate an idea about what causes what. A clinician
should be able to describe evidence from direct observations and inter-

view information that supports or refutes the hypothesis. For example, a clinician who suspects that parent–child conflict is a primary family-level factor contributing to an adolescent's suicidal thoughts should be able to describe concrete examples of parent–child conflict that precede the suicide threats. Similarly, the therapist should identify whether the youth's suicidal thoughts occur even when parent–child conflicts do not, and whether there are times when parent–child conflicts occur but suicidal threats do not. If parent–child conflicts are chronic, but suicidal threats are intermittent, then evidence that parent–child conflict is a primary driver of suicidal thoughts is relatively weak.

Initially, hypotheses should pertain to the most proximal causes of behavior. *Proximal causes* are interactions and events in everyday living that seem to be directly connected with the problem behavior. Among everyday interactions between caregivers and their children, teachers and students, peer groups, and so on, MST therapists identify particular sequences of interaction that seem to precede and follow the occurrence of a particular problem. For example, lack of monitoring is often one proximal cause of runaway behavior. As depicted in Figure 2.2, the factors that contribute to lack of monitoring vary from family to family. In one family, the factors may include the parents' long work hours, marital problems, and lack of knowledge about parenting. In another family, a single parent may have the necessary knowledge and skills to parent but suffers from depression and lacks the social support needed to parent effectively. In both families, the parent's discipline style is a direct and proximal cause of the runaway behavior. The work hours, marital problems, depression, and so on have an indirect or more distal effect on the youth's running away, but a direct or more proximal effect on the parent's monitoring practices.

Hypotheses are generally tested by evaluating the effects of interventions derived from a hypothesis. For example, if interventions designed to decrease the use of harsh punishment were implemented and measurable decreases in runaway incidents followed, the team would have some evidence to support the hypothesis that harsh discipline strategies were direct contributors to the child's running away. Similarly (see Figure 2.2), if interventions to address conflicting parenting styles enabled the parents to monitor their child more consistently, the team would have evidence that these more distal factors were directly related to the monitoring and indirectly related to the child's running away. Alternatively, if the parent's ineffective discipline practices did not change as conflicting parenting decreased and monitoring increased, then the therapist would identify other possible drivers of the ineffective discipline practices. Or, if the child continued to run away even after monitoring practices increased, the therapist would identify other proximal drivers of runaway incidents. The process of developing hypotheses regarding factors that contribute to a particular problem (or treatment gain), gathering evidence to support or refute the hypotheses, designing and implementing interventions to test the hypotheses, and developing new hypotheses on the basis of the intervention outcomes is ongoing and recursive.

## Intermediary Treatment Goals

Following the initial conceptualization of factors contributing to referral, the therapist and team identify intermediary treatment goals. Such goals should be achievable in the short term and reflect direct movement toward the achievement of overarching goals. Intermediary goals should (1) be logically linked to overarching goals, (2) address factors in the systemic context hypothesized to contribute to the referral problems, and (3) be achievable over a period of days or weeks. Often, several intermediary goals related to a single overarching goal are pursued simultaneously, as the systems and interactions they target reciprocally influence one another. At other times, intermediary goals may need to be pursued in sequential order.

With the intermediary goals defined, the treatment team next identifies the range of treatment modalities and techniques that might be effective toward meeting the intermediary goals and tailors these to the specific strengths and weaknesses of the targeted client system (e.g., marital, parent–child, family–school). Interventions are generally designed by the MST therapist in consultation with caregivers, and implemented primarily by the caregivers and other key figures in the youth's ecology (e.g., teachers, relatives, coaches, the parents of peers, etc.). Thus, at any point in treatment a therapist may be helping a mother to monitor her 15-year-old daughter's intake of antidepressant medication; soliciting help from parents of peers who harbor the daughter when she runs away from home; negotiating an arrangement with teachers to establish a daily attendance and behavior reporting mechanism; helping a stepfather, mother, and daughter reduce the verbal and physical aggression between the daughter and stepfather that precipitates runaway behavior; and soliciting relatives' help in enacting a safety plan when the daughter verbalizes suicidal thoughts.

## Intervention Development and Implementation

MST intervention strategies are designed to address prioritized "fit factors," consistent with the nine MST principles, and drawn from empirically supported treatment approaches for youth and families identified earlier in this chapter. Descriptions of family, peer, school, social support, individual, and crisis stabilization interventions used in MST are provided in subsequent chapters of this book. These descriptions illustrate how empirically supported treatment approaches are integrated to address the unique strengths and weaknesses in the social ecology of each youth and his or her family. Creativity on the part of intervention participants (e.g., caregivers, teachers, etc.), the clinician, and the clinical team is an important element of the process of tailoring an empirically supported intervention to these strengths and weaknesses.

To increase the likelihood of intervention success, interventions should be accurately targeted, well specified, and completely and correctly implemented. An *accurately targeted intervention* is one that addresses one or more prioritized fit factors. A *well-specified intervention* is one that makes clear what each pertinent participant in the social ecology will do, and when and how he or she will do it. In the case of Jennifer, for example, after progress was made addressing some proximal drivers of conflict between Jennifer and Mary, such as inappropriate stepfamily expectations and conflicting parenting styles, John suggested that conflict would be further reduced if Jennifer and Mary spent more "quality time" together. "Quality time" together was operationally defined as 30 minutes of shopping in the mall without any of the younger children or John present. To implement an intervention completely, participants must have the skills, practice, and contextual support to implement the intervention. To this end, MST clinicians routinely model an intervention, provide opportunities for participants to practice the intervention in role plays, and observe when the intervention is implemented for the first time and subsequently if it appears the intervention is not working. To arrange for a successful 30 minutes of shopping time at the mall, for example, Mary and Jennifer had to agree in advance on a day for the date, John or Jennifer's grandmother had to baby-sit for the younger children, and Jennifer had to be on her Ritalin.

As interventions are implemented and their success is monitored, barriers to favorable outcomes may become evident at several levels, as described next.

### Identifying and Overcoming Barriers to Progress

In spite of significant efforts, interventions with children and families presenting serious clinical problems often fail. Clinicians and supervisors are encouraged to examine the reasons for failure (i.e., barriers to change). In light of information obtained about the barriers, aspects of interventions are changed. Common barriers to intervention success include:

- Faulty or incomplete conceptualizations of the fit of the problem targeted for a particular intervention.
- Intermediary goals that do not reflect the most powerful and proximal predictors of the target behavior, such that interventions designed to achieve these goals miss the mark.
- Appropriate intermediary goals, but interventions that do not follow logically from the goals.
- Failure of the clinician to implement the intervention correctly or completely, or to ensure that the individuals (e.g., parent, grandparent, teacher) who were to implement the intervention had sufficient understanding and competency to do so.

Each of these factors, in turn, may be influenced by a combination of case-specific, clinician-specific, and supervision-specific issues. That is, at any juncture of MST, it may be helpful—indeed necessary—to consider not only the details of the particular case, but the extent to which the clinician, the team, and the supervisor are engaging in the behaviors necessary to help families achieve their treatment goals. Thus, the MST treatment process is self-reflexive for clinicians and supervisors, who continuously consider their own behavior as factors that contribute to intervention success and failure.

## DELIVERING MST: A HOME-BASED MODEL OF SERVICE DELIVERY

MST has been provided within a home-based model of service delivery in community-based clinical trials and community-initiated programs around the country. Intensive home-based services have increasingly been recommended as desirable alternatives to the use of restrictive and expensive placements for youth with serious behavioral and emotional problems. A basic assumption underlying most programs is that children are better off being raised in their natural families than in surrogate families or institutions (Nelson & Landsman, 1992). Thus, the family is seen as a source of strengths, even when serious and multiple needs are evident, and a common objective is to empower families to meet their needs in the future. To date, however, few home-based programs have delivered evidence-based treatments to youth and their families (Fraser, Nelson, & Rivard, 1997; Henegan, Horwitz, & Leventhal, 1997).

The intent of using a home-based model to deliver MST is to provide very intensive clinical interventions when and where they are needed to alter the youth's natural ecology in ways that will avert imminent and future out-of-home placements. A number of program practices described in the MST organizational manual (Strother, Swenson, & Schoenwald, 1998) are designed to support therapists and supervisors in meeting these objectives. Specifically, the following practices are recommended:

- MST therapists are full-time master's-level, or highly competent, clinically skilled, bachelor's-level, professionals assigned to the MST program solely.
- MST therapists operate in teams of no fewer than two and no more than four therapists, plus a supervisor.
- MST caseloads do not exceed six families per therapist, with the normal range being three or four "active" cases.
- Expected duration of treatment is 3–5 months.
- MST therapists are accessible at times that are convenient for their clients and, in times of crisis, very quickly.
- The MST program will have a 24-hour-per-day, 7-day-per-week on-call system to provide coverage when MST therapists are on vacation or taking personal time.

The home-based model of service delivery removes common barriers to service access such as transportation, inconvenient appointment times, and need for childcare. Removing such barriers to access often enhances the family's engagement in the treatment process. In addition, low caseloads and flexible hours allow therapists to expend intensive and sustained effort when such is needed.

The duration and frequency of treatment sessions vary in accordance with changing circumstances, needs, and treatment progress. Sessions generally occur less frequently when evidence indicates family members and others in the natural ecology are increasingly able to manage the youth's problems effectively. For example, a therapist may stay with a family from the end of the school day until bedtime every day when first helping a caregiver and adolescent decrease volatile parent–child conflicts that occur during that time. The therapist would decrease the frequency of visits and length of stay when evidence indicates the conflicts occur less frequently, are less intense, and can be managed by the parent, child, and other family members.

Moreover, the home-based model of service delivery enhances the ecological validity of assessment and intervention activities. Therapists observe and try to help change behaviors where they naturally occur rather than in an artificial setting such as a clinic. Thus, intervention strategies are tailored to the specific circumstances in which they are to be implemented by family members and others in the youth's social ecology, thereby increasing the likelihood that treatment gains will be maintained after MST ends.

## CONCLUSION

The nine MST principles and the MST analytic process enable therapists to understand, prioritize, and address the complex realities facing children with serious emotional disturbance and their families. The MST principles are consistent with social-ecological theory and empirical evidence regarding the etiology and treatment of behavioral and emotional problems. The analytic process specifies steps for identifying the likely causes of problems, developing interventions to address them, evaluating the impact of the interventions, identifying barriers to intervention success, and adjusting intervention strategies accordingly. As such, the analytic process is designed to stimulate "scientific thinking"—hypothesis development and testing—about the causes of and solutions to problems among therapists, caregivers, and others in the youth's ecology who implement interventions. Random acts of intervention are therefore minimized, and the likelihood of rapid treatment progress and sustainability of treatment gains is increased.

# CHAPTER 3

# Family Interventions and Building Indigenous Family Supports

Building and sustaining effective caregiver and family functioning is vital to achieving favorable child outcomes. This chapter describes important determinants of caregiver and family functioning and interventions that can be effective at ameliorating family-related difficulties associated with these determinants. In addition, the chapter explains why the development of indigenous family support systems is critical to the sustainability of favorable change among family members.

Families come in many forms across many cultures: two biological or adoptive parents, one biological parent and one stepparent, a single parent who is divorced or who has never been married, one or more grandparents or other relatives acting in the parental role. Divorced, remarried, and/or never-married parents raise increased numbers of children in the United States (U.S. Bureau of the Census, 1995). Regardless of the particular form a family takes, core functions of the family include protecting family members and providing them with economic support; offering education and religious or spiritual training; providing affection and recreation for members; and defining a role in the larger community (Emery, 1999). Subsumed within these broad functions are the many and often changing tasks associated with socializing children.

## FOCI OF MST FAMILY INTERVENTIONS: RISK AND PROTECTIVE FACTORS

Multisystemic conceptualizations of family functioning are guided by social-ecological, family systems, and social learning theories and the research that supports them. Research on child development, developmental psychopathology, marital relations, and individual parent and child characteristics associated with positive and negative outcomes for youth has identified numerous family risk and protective factors. These factors fall into several general categories, including (1) interactions among family members, (2) parenting practices, (3) the marital relationship (or its proxy), (4) characteristics of the individual caregiver, (5) the social support and concrete resources (e.g., housing, transportation) available to the caregiver and family, and (6) characteristics of the child. The ongoing MST assessment of family functioning is directed toward identifying which particular combination of these factors contributes to a referral problem and/or can be used as levers for change.

### The Family as a System

MST perspectives on family functioning embody systems theories and the assumptions of multicausality and reciprocity of interactions that characterize these theories. Thus, the behavior of all family members is understood in terms of ongoing and repetitive patterns of family transactions rather than in terms of unidirectional and linear interpersonal or intrapsychic processes. Problems are seen as both affecting and being affected by how the family interacts as a whole. The present-focused and solution-oriented nature of MST is particularly consonant with strategic (Haley, 1976), social learning (Patterson, 1982), and structural (Minuchin, 1974) approaches to family interventions. Central to these approaches is the view that families have organized ways of behaving, and that careful observation of family interactions will reveal recurrent patterns that sustain a particular problem or set of problems. According to Haley (1976) these "recursive sequences" of behavior often occur in "chains of three or more interactions" (p. 105) involving more than two people. Thus, the relatively simple task of detecting whether $A$ causes $B$, gives way to the more complex task of detecting that $A$ causes $B$ which triggers $C$ in a way that amplifies or changes the impact of $A$ on $B$.

Research on risk and protective factors for a variety of externalizing and internalizing problems in children and adolescents is consistent with the notion that recurrent interaction patterns among family members can contribute to problem behavior (Mash, 1998). For example, risk factors for depression and anxiety include parent–child interactions that inadvertently reinforce anxious or depressive responses (Mash, 1998; Ollendick & King, 1998); family conflict has been associated with a variety of problems in youths (Foster & Robbins, 1998); and repetitive cycles of aversive interaction among parents, children, and siblings contribute to the development of antisocial behavior (Patterson, 1982; Patterson & Reid, 1984). In addition to familywide interaction patterns, some risk factors are specific to interactions in the parent–child subsystem, others to the marital subsystem or relations between adult heads of a family even if they are not marital partners.

## Parenting Practices

In studies of risk factors for child and adolescent behavior problems, the aspects of parenting most consistently implicated are inconsistent and harsh discipline, inadequate parental monitoring, parent–child conflict, and low affective bonding (Cicchetti & Toth, 1995; Henggeler, 1997b). Research on normative child development indicates that four broad parenting styles are associated with differential outcomes for children. Each of the four styles entails varying degrees of parental warmth, control, and involvement. The styles are known as authoritative, authoritarian, permissive, and neglectful (Baumrind, 1989).

*Authoritative* (high control, high warmth) parents are responsive to the reasonable needs and desires of the child, but also make maturity demands appropriate to the child's stage of development. Parents have clear and well-defined expectations and rules regarding the child's school performance, participation in household chores, and interpersonal behavior with family members, peers, and adults and authority figures outside the home (e.g., teachers, other relatives, neighbors, coaches, etc.). Authoritative parenting is associated with a range of positive outcomes, such as positive academic achievement, social responsibility, and positive peer relationships.

*Authoritarian* (high control, low warmth) parents are directive and overcontrolling, and require their children to have an unquestioning obedience to parental authority. When a child deviates from parental rules, punishment tends to be severe and is often physical. When teaching the child new skills, behaviors, or tasks, the authoritarian parent is directive, giving direct verbal orders and often physically taking over the activity being taught. Thus, the child rarely participates in making choices and decisions, and therefore has little opportunity to grapple with the consequences of his or her own choices and decisions.

*Permissive* (high warmth, low control) parents provide their children with little structure and discipline, make few demands for mature behavior, and tolerate even those impulses in children that meet with societal disapproval. Permissive parents are typically warm and responsive, but not demanding.

*Neglectful* (low warmth, low control) parents offer little affection or discipline to their children and appear to have little concern for or interest in parenting. That is, neglectful parents are neither responsive to the reasonable needs and desires of the youth, nor demanding of responsible, age-appropriate behavior with respect to tasks or interpersonal relationships.

Of the four parenting types, authoritarian and permissive parenting are most strongly related to externalizing problems such as aggression and substance abuse, whereas neglectful parenting is most strongly related to children's distress, including symptoms of depression (Luthar, 1999; Steinberg, Lamborn, Darling, Mounts, & Dornbusch, 1994).

Parenting practices are generally both stable and variable. Consistent with the constructs of reciprocity and contextuality central to social-ecological theory, however, research indicates that parental behavior varies somewhat in accordance with a child's age, family circumstances, and across children in the same family (Holden & Miller, 1999). Finally, there are multiple determinants of a parenting style (e.g., permissive parenting) or of a particular practice or problem (e.g., lack of monitoring). For some caregivers, a combination of work schedule, marital problems, and depression might contribute to permissive practices; for others, lack of knowledge about effective discipline practices, social isolation, and fear that setting limits will escalate parent–child conflict do so. One schematic tool often used by MST clinicians to identify the factors that influence a particular parent–child dyad is illustrated in Figure 3.1. MST intervention strategies are individualized to address the particular combination of individual parent, intrafamilial, and extrafamilial factors that contribute to ineffective parenting practices.

## Relations among Coparenting Adults

When two adults head families, the relationship between those adults has considerable impact on the functioning of all family members. The adults may be the married biological parents, grandparents, other kin of all children in the household, or a couple in which one or both parents are stepparents to some children in the household. The adults may be married to one another or not, previously married or not. In some fami-

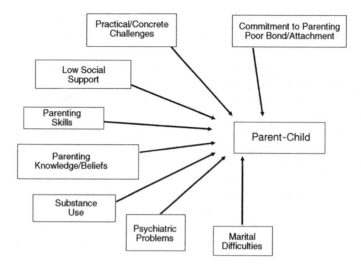

**FIGURE 3.1.** Barriers to effective parenting.

lies headed by a single parent, the responsibilities of parenting are shared with another family member, such as a grandparent. In any of these scenarios, effective parenting requires adults who share parenting responsibilities to be consistent in their expectations, limit setting, discipline strategies, and affective investment in the children. Many factors can interfere with interparental consistency, including concrete obstacles such as mutually exclusive work hours or financial problems, different parenting styles, lack of knowledge or skill about effective parenting practices, or parental depression or substance abuse. Sometimes, however, problems in the adult relationship itself interfere with effective parenting.

For couples who are married or living together in a committed relationship, partners generally need to love and feel loved, to honor their commitment to monogamy, and to experience the relationship as one in which they get at least as much as they give. Chronic conflict between partners can arise on any of these fronts. Research shows that such conflict is associated with externalizing problems in children and adolescents, depression in mothers, inconsistent parenting, and increased parent–child conflict. Similarly, when a parent and grandparent or other relative share the parenting role, conflict about a range of issues not limited to parenting has been shown to contribute to stress and depression in the adults and compromised parenting practices (Chase-Lansdale, Brooks-Gunn, & Zamsky, 1994). When individuals remarry, the challenges of parenting one's own and/or another's children while laying the foundations for a new marital relationship can overwhelm the new marriage.

Thus, MST therapists assess the nature of relations between adult heads of households to determine whether and how strengths and weaknesses in those relations contribute to referral problems or to barriers to treatment progress. When the heads of families live in different households, therapists must assess the strengths and weaknesses of the multiple adult dyads that could influence a child's behavior, and vice versa (how the child's behavior influences the adults' relations). Thus, for example, 14-year-old Kendra lived with her mother and stepfather of 3 years during the week and with her father and his wife on weekends. To establish the consistent medication monitoring and contingencies needed to manage Kendra's ADHD symptoms and oppositional behavior, the therapist had to address conflicts within the currently married couples and between the ex-spouses (Kendra's biological parents).

## Individual Caregiver Factors

Individuals who experience depression, anxiety, or more serious psychiatric disturbances often have difficulty executing parenting tasks effectively. Much of the research in this area focuses on mothers. Depressed mothers tend to be less attentive than other mothers to their children, express more negative affect, make more negative attributions about their children, vacillate between intrusive and disengaged behaviors, and are at risk for hostile, coercive parenting and child maltreatment (Cicchetti & Toth, 1995). Similarly, parental substance abuse is consistently linked with problematic parenting practices, including poor attentiveness to cues and communication with younger children, and use of authoritarian parenting styles that reinforce negative attention-seeking behavior with older children (Mayes & Bornstein, 1997). Although others often view mothers who abuse substances as uncaring parents, many of them are deeply concerned about their children and strongly invested in improving their life circumstances (Luthar & Suchman, 2000). Importantly, mental disorders and alcohol or drug use frequently co-occur. Finally, commitment to parenting may be compromised for some parents with psychiatric or substance abuse problems. Lack of commitment can also occur, however, when a solid affective bond between parent and child has never been developed or has been seriously compromised by frequent separations (e.g., child placements or custody changes; relocation, hospitalization, or imprisonment of a parent) or exceptionally chronic and intense parent–child conflict.

## Social Support and Concrete Resources

The final sections of this chapter focus on helping families to build the indigenous supports needed to effectively manage the inevitable challenges of raising children and the added challenges that can arise when youngsters have chronic psychiatric conditions (e.g., ADHD, depression, bipolar disorder, etc.). The availability of high-quality support from family, friends, coworkers, neighbors, and community organizations is strongly associated with the capacity of families to function effectively and respond to changes in circumstances (Reiss & Price, 1996). Social support is consistently linked with positive marital adjustment, effective management of parent–child problems, and a host of other positive family outcomes (Pierce, Sarason, & Sarason, 1995), even among the most economically disadvantaged families (Luthar, 1999). Conversely, when parents or grandparents serving in a parental role are socially isolated, they engage in less responsive and more harsh and ineffective parenting practices. Social isolation also exacerbates depression and other psychiatric conditions. Friends, relatives, and neighbors can help families overcome or cope with concrete obstacles such as lack of transportation, overcrowded living conditions, and financial difficulties. Sometimes, however, the resources required to overcome concrete obstacles exceed the capacity of even a strong social support system, and formal assistance from one or more agencies (e.g., public housing authority, public transportation voucher scholarships, community heating banks, etc.) is required.

## FAMILY-FOCUSED INTERVENTIONS

MST family interventions draw extensively upon behavioral, cognitive-behavioral, strategic, and structural family therapies. Interventions may range from simple, focused behavioral interventions such as establishing a tracking chart for compliance with scheduled Ritalin doses to a more complex series of interventions that simultaneously address parent–child conflict, parental substance abuse, and social isolation of the family.

### Building Caregiver "Buy-In"

Children with serious emotional disturbance have often been examined, diagnosed, treated, and placed out of the home by multiple mental health professionals. Their caregivers often feel poorly served, if not blamed, by such professionals. Caregivers may be frustrated with the challenges of trying to manage their child's behavioral and emotional problems, and some have come to believe that they can have no positive impact on the child's difficulties. The notion that changed parenting practices may facilitate more effective youth functioning may therefore come as a surprise, if not an affront, to some caregivers. MST therapists should avoid unnecessary confrontation with caregivers, while ensuring that they understand the importance of change. In some instances, pointing out the negative consequences of current parenting practices for the life of the caregiver (e.g., explosive confrontations at home, frequent absence from work to deal with the child's crises, aversive interactions with school personnel, etc.) is more effective initially than pointing out the negative consequences of such practices for the youth. For others, pointing out the long-term negative consequences for the child is more salient. In any case, the therapist must be able to convince a caregiver that a change of parenting practice is needed before attempting change. The therapist may need to enlist the support of family members or friends respected by the parent to accomplish this task. Throughout the process, the practitioner generally should provide emotional support to the caregiver and highlight any positive aspects of parenting (Principle 2) while assessing family factors that might be linked with identified problems.

## Changing Parenting Practices

When it becomes clear that a child's problems are maintained by permissive, authoritarian, or neglectful parenting styles, the clinician and the caregiver together identify factors that might be sustaining the ineffective practice or style. Working with the strengths and needs of the caregiver, the family, and the social ecology, the clinician tailors interventions to address these factors and enhance the effectiveness of parenting practices. Areas often targeted for change include discipline strategies and monitoring of the youth. When one caregiver heads a household, consistency in parenting behavior along these lines is key to the effectiveness of changed parenting practices. When households are headed by more than one adult, the clinician helps ensure consistency of practice between the adults.

### CHANGING DISCIPLINE STRATEGIES

When it becomes apparent that a child's difficulties are being maintained in part by a caregiver's discipline strategies, the MST practitioner has three general tasks in providing caregivers with alternative strategies. The therapist must help caregivers to (1) set clearly defined rules for the child's behavior, (2) develop sets of consequences that are inextricably linked to the rules, and (3) effectively monitor a child's compliance or noncompliance with rules, even when the child is not in the caregiver's presence. Richard Munger has detailed many of the steps involved in accomplishing the three tasks listed above in a book entitled *Changing Children's Behavior Quickly* (1993). MST practitioners have often found this book useful when teaching caregivers more effective methods of handling behavior problems. The MST manual for treatment of antisocial behavior (Henggeler et al., 1998) reprises these steps in some detail. To summarize, MST therapists should be prepared to help caregivers develop and enforce *rules* that define desired and undesired behaviors in objective and measurable terms and that are enforced 100% of the time in an unemotional way. *Privileges* should be dispensed or withheld in accordance with the child's compliance or noncompliance with the rules. These privileges should be developmentally appropriate, valued by the child, and able to be managed by the adults without threatening basic necessities such as shelter, food (for sustenance vs. snacks or treats), everyday clothing (vs. the latest fad item), and love. Therapists should prepare caregivers to discuss the nature of the rules and privileges with their children before the structure is implemented. Children and adolescents should understand what is changing, what will be expected of them, and what to expect from their caregivers when strategies designed to change their behavior are put in place. Modifying the cognitive expectations of children and adolescents can expedite desired changes in behavior. When two or more adults are raising a child, the adults must develop rules and sequences jointly and enforce them consistently.

## ADULT MONITORING

Related to effective discipline is appropriate monitoring of a youth's activities, whereabouts, and social contacts. Parental awareness of a youngster's behavior at home, at school, and in the community is necessary to develop discipline strategies that reinforce appropriate behaviors and discourage inappropriate behaviors in multiple settings. Because increased independence from caregivers is developmentally appropriate for adolescents, however, establishing necessary and sufficient monitoring strategies can be challenging. Moreover, when a youngster experiences psychiatric problems that increases risk of harm to him- or herself or to others, vigilant monitoring of safety and compliance with prescribed medication is also necessary. Common barriers to effective monitoring include lack of knowledge about risks a youth faces outside the home (e.g., a parent may not know that a close peer is depressed or suicidal or that prescribed medications are discarded at school), scheduling challenges created by long and often inflexible work hours, the demands of caring for multiple children, and social isolation. Also, any of the factors that can impact discipline strategies (e.g., psychiatric conditions, substance abuse, poor health, marital problems) can also interfere with effective monitoring and should be addressed if this is the case.

Whereas parents are the primary sources of structure, limit setting, and discipline, they will often require the help of relatives, teachers, the parents of the youngster's peers, and neighbors for monitoring efforts. Clinicians may need to help caregivers to establish effective "working relationships" with individuals who can observe and report on their child's activities. For example, neighbors might take turns monitoring the school bus stop, if that is where fights break out or if some riders head toward a known drug-dealing corner when they get off the bus. Or an aunt who works the swing shift may be asked to stop at the home of her nephew on the way to work each day to ensure that he comes directly home from school. All such arrangements require a certain level of mutuality. The parent who benefits from the aunt's afterschool spot-check on her son might invite the aunt to dinner on a weekend or run a needed errand for her. The extent to which such "quid pro quo" arrangements are formalized varies in accordance with the intimacy of the relationships and consistency with which more or less formally structured arrangements must be executed to achieve the desired results.

## Increasing Chances for Success

The therapist should prepare caregivers for the likelihood that their child or adolescent will react negatively to changes in their parenting practices. In anticipation of the child's testing of changed practices, the therapist supports the caregiver in "sticking with" the program and finding support for appropriate parenting from other adults (e.g., spouse, relatives, other parents) in the natural environment (Principle 9). Permissive parents are particularly likely to need support when their children test new rules. Such parents sometimes feel they would rather live with the child's frustrating, worrisome, or obnoxious behavior than with the negative reaction the child displays in response to new rules. When the behavior in question gives rise to a "predictable" crisis (e.g., threats to run away, engage in self-injurious behavior, physically harm a family member), specific and comprehensive steps are taken to help prepare caregivers and their support system to manage the crisis. The development of safety plans for predictable crises and for management of crises once they have occurred is described in Chapter 5.

## Anticipating Testing

In many cases, a child or adolescent who is testing new parenting practices may display increased irritability, verbal aggression, threats of physical aggression against self or others, or property-damaging physical aggression (e.g., breaking furniture, punching a hole in the wall). Therapists must help caregivers to recognize that the consequences of giving in are likely to extend beyond their home and negatively affect their child. The example of Rachel illustrates this dilemma.

Rachel was a depressed 14-year-old girl whose verbal suicide threats had prompted two 72-hour emergency hospitalizations for psychiatric evaluations prior to referral for MST. In the year prior to referral, Rachel had been truant from school often and had begun experimenting with drugs and slipping into a deviant peer group. Rachel's grandmother, Ms. Clarke, had been her primary caregiver for 4 years prior to the referral. Ms. Clarke's parenting style was permissive; she was reluctant to establish rules and consequences for Rachel about school attendance and peer activities. Factors contributing to her reluctance were lack of knowledge and skill about implementing rules and consequences; lack of support from other adults for enforcement of new practices; and fear that Rachel would perceive such behavior as a signal that Ms. Clarke did not care about her, which, in turn, might deepen Rachel's depression.

The therapist first tried to remedy the knowledge, skill, and social support barriers, thinking that Ms. Clarke's concerns about her relationship with Rachel and exacerbating the depression might abate when she felt capable of implementing rules and consequences effectively. Ms. Clarke agreed, and expressed interest in learning to establish rules and consequences and getting support from her sister. As Ms. Clarke practiced setting rules and consequences in role-played sessions with the therapist, she worried aloud that Rachel would perceive her as cruel and unkind, that their warm relationship would end, and that Rachel would become suicidal as a result. The therapist tried to help Ms. Clarke to understand that, although Rachel might indeed be upset by the new rules and consequences, the lack of rules and consequences contributed to her lack of school success and her increased drug use, both of which had been shown to exacerbate Rachel's depression. This reminder was not intended as a scare tactic (which would violate the principles of MST), but was intended to help the grandmother understand the linkages between her behavior and Rachel's chances to succeed at school and in the community despite her depression.

## MATTER-OF-FACT IMPLEMENTATION OF NEW PRACTICES

Caregivers should try to enforce rules in an unemotional way. They should avoid badgering the child or adolescent to follow the rules, and allow the decision regarding compliance to be made by the child. If rules are well written, there should be little argument about whether the rules were followed. Moreover, caregivers are more likely to enforce rules if punishments provide some payoff to themselves. In any case, the caregiver should not respond to the child's attempts to argue about this issue. This may be particularly difficult when the behavior presents a threat to the safety of the child or others, as was the case with Rachel. The therapist helped Ms. Clarke manage her understandable worry and distress when Rachel issued tearful complaints that the new rules signaled Ms. Clarke's lack of caring about her. From observing these interactions, the therapist had ample evidence that when Ms. Clarke responded to Rachel's complaints with protestations that she did care, and noted that she was worried about Rachel becoming more depressed, Rachel's testing behavior increased. Thus, the therapist stayed with Ms. Clarke for her first attempts, and together they coached Ms. Clarke's sister to help her stand firm. Because caregivers are not often aware that their understandably angry, worried, or otherwise emotional responses may reinforce the very behavior they are trying to attenuate, therapists may have to provide the evidence that this is the case, and then help caregivers to manage their responses accordingly.

## ADDRESSING FACTORS THAT CONTRIBUTE TO INEFFECTIVE PARENTING PRACTICES

As noted earlier, the extent to which a particular caregiver can alter her or his parenting practices is often influenced by a combination of the factors shown in Figure 3.1. If these factors are not taken into account when interventions to alter parenting practices are initially designed, they may emerge as barriers to intervention success. Thus, in the initial design of parenting interventions and when trying to understand why an intervention may have failed, the clinician and team should examine the following potential barriers to successful outcome.

### Knowledge, Beliefs, and Skills

Numerous studies have demonstrated associations between parental knowledge, beliefs, and skills and child outcomes. Knowledge regarding child development (e.g., at what age can children anticipate the future, think abstractly) and beliefs about the motivations of children's behavior (e.g., that it is always willful) have been associated with irritable, harsh parenting practices and with conduct disorder and aggression in children. Similarly, cognitive distortions in both parents and children are associated with family conflict (Robin, Bedway, & Gilroy, 1994). In assessing the role of knowledge and beliefs in maintaining ineffective parenting practices, practitioners should attend to parental language signaling unrealistic expectations about their child's capacities and motivations, and should collect evidence regarding the correspondence between these beliefs and caregiver behavior. This evidence is often needed to develop a rationale compelling enough to engage the caregiver in the process of changing long-held beliefs.

When evidence indicates that parental misconceptions or faulty beliefs are helping to sustain ineffective parenting practices, the practitioner should attempt to understand the bases for the beliefs prior to making attempts to change them. For example, a father's continued use of harsh physical punishment in response to the impulsive behavior of a 10-year-old boy with ADHD may be associated with two beliefs: (1) that the behavior is willful and (2) that such punishment was effective on him when he was a child. With respect to the first belief, it may be helpful to explain the nature of ADHD and to present the evidence that the boy may have the disorder. With respect to beliefs developed on the basis of a caregiver's childhood experiences, we have rarely found it useful to dispute the caregiver's stance, appeal to changing times, or cite facts and figures about the deleterious effects of harsh physical punishment. Instead, we often point out ways in which this particular child is experiencing difficulties (e.g., school failure, suspensions, or expulsions; mood swings; irritability) that may warrant alternative, perhaps even unusual, approaches to discipline. Such a strategy may increase parental receptivity to the idea that his or her behavior may need to be modified to benefit this unique child. By focusing on the caregiver's ability to help the child and on the long-term negative consequences of the youth's present behavior, the practitioner is more likely to elicit parental cooperation in treatment.

Cognitive distortions on the part of both caregiver and youth often contribute to caregiver–child conflict. A caregiver may believe that children should respond with absolute obedience, while a teen is convinced that her caregiver's limit setting will ruin her life. To assist families in changing distortions that contribute to the fit of an identified problem targeted for MST treatment, the practitioner may reframe the distorted cognitions and help family members identify various aspects of unreasonable thinking. Thus, for example, Mr. Smith's hotly contested efforts to set an age-appropriate curfew for his 15-year-old son, Steven, could be described (reframed) as arising out of concern for Steven's safety and well-being, rather than as a deliberate attempt to control Steven's every move. To develop a more objective understanding about what motivates the behavior of a parent or child, the therapist may need to teach more effective communication (e.g., listening, stating the problem in non-blaming terms) and interpersonal problem-solving skills to one or more family members. In addition, interventions that monitor and test the validity of faulty beliefs are often necessary. Steven might be asked to list specifically how his life will be ruined by a curfew, and relevant observers (e.g., Steven, Mr. Smith, a teacher) would monitor how frequently those things occurred within a week and what consequences ensued. More often than not, the ruinous consequences anticipated by the youth or parent do not come to pass (i.e., the cognitions are distortions). The therapist helps the youth and caregiver to recognize when beliefs are not confirmed by experience and designs interventions that support more accurate appraisals. For example, if Steven's curfew had prevented him from attending a valued extracurricular event, the therapist might model for Mr. Smith how to interrupt Steven's predictable complaint that his life had been ruined and how to acknowledge that Steven was disappointed about missing the event without "giving in." The therapist would also point out that missing the event did not lead to rejection from peers—the dire consequence predicted by Steven. The therapist would help Mr. Smith either to ignore or to interrupt Steven's complaints calmly, depending upon which was more effective. Together, they might also bootstrap the curfew intervention to specify circumstances, if any, under which exceptions could be earned or granted.

Methods used to increase parental knowledge and skills are geared to the clinician's assessment of the amount of teaching, role play, live practice, and practitioner involvement needed by a particular caregiver to understand and implement new parenting strategies. Lay-friendly books and manuals on child development, a particular child behavior problem such as ADHD, or parenting tips can be legitimate sources of information if they are based on sound science. MST therapists rarely use "bibliotherapy," however. Research indicates that reading about parenting, or even attending classes on parenting, is generally not helpful to the caregivers of children with serious problems. Moreover, the multiple demands these caregivers face often preclude the availability of quiet reading time, and language barriers (e.g., not fluent in English, literacy problems) exist for some caregivers. Thus, therapists tailor information about relevant (i.e., to achieve a treatment goal) developmental, diagnostic, or parenting issues to the venues most likely to be understood by a particular caregiver. In the case of the father who used physical punishment with his son with ADHD, the therapist might explain the nature of

ADHD and offer to type a short list of hallmark symptoms for the father to discuss with the team psychiatrist. For a parent–teen dyad whose heated conflicts are predictable to the therapist, but not to the dyad, the interactions might be audiotaped and played back in a session during which the therapist identifies the cues that the conflict will begin or escalate. However new information is delivered, the therapist must ensure that caregivers understand and can use the information. Thus, a therapist might describe the cognitive capacities of the average 9-year-old to help a grandparent understand that more frequent rewards are needed to change the child's behavior. The therapist and the grandparent must then craft specific plans for increasing the frequency of rewards and monitoring their dispensation based on the child's behavior.

### Individual Psychiatric Problems

When the practitioner suspects that a caregiver is experiencing depression, anxiety, or a more serious *psychiatric disturbance,* several steps should be taken. First, the practitioner should obtain information regarding the intensity, severity, and duration of the problem from the parent, other family members, and, as appropriate, professionals who may have treated the parent. This information is needed to determine the extent to which (1) the psychiatric problem contributes to the referral problem or presents a barrier to change, (2) the psychiatric disorder can be safely and effectively addressed by the MST team, and (3) periodic or ongoing collaboration with a psychiatrist may be required to ensure safe and effective pharmacological treatment for the parent.

To understand the fit between the psychiatric disturbance of a caregiver and identified child problems, and vice versa, the practitioner observes interactions within and between systems (Principle 5). One of the interaction sequences that contributed to the referral of Michael Calhoun for psychiatric hospitalization provides a relevant example. Michael had been psychiatrically hospitalized on an emergency basis before being referred to the MST team. Ms. Calhoun, who had both social phobia and depression, became particularly anxious and hopeless when she received phone calls or notes from school personnel asking her to meet with them about Michael's behavior at school. As Ms. Calhoun's anxiety increased, so did her avoidance of school contact. Meanwhile, school personnel, unaware of Ms. Calhoun's psychiatric difficulties, increased their telephone and written requests to meet with her. These requests further exacerbated Ms. Calhoun's anxiety, which prompted her to frantically confront Michael about his behavior at school. Michael consistently responded with anger and agitation. Their ensuing arguments escalated to the point at which Michael threatened his mother with a knife.

Consistent with all aspects of assessment in MST, when the psychiatric problem of a caregiver is shown to impact a referral problem or treatment progress, the individual and social-ecological factors that contribute to the problem or interfere with effective management of its symptoms should be delineated. Many psychiatric problems (e.g., depression, bipolar disorder, anxiety disorders) can be managed effectively with a combination of medication, cognitive-behavioral interventions, and well-specified and consistently implemented family and social support strategies. Chronic stresses such as marital or family problems, financial problems, social isolation, and poor health can contribute to psychiatric problems; conversely, alleviation or effective management of such stresses can help attenuate psychiatric symptoms. Cognitive factors (e.g., attribution biases, all-or-nothing thinking) also play a role in some disorders. Finally, changes in circumstances (e.g., recent loss of job, death in the family, change in medication regimen, traumatic experiences) can exacerbate conditions that are typically well managed.

## DEPRESSION

Because depression is reported fairly frequently among caregivers of youth with serious behavioral and emotional problems, clinicians should be able to implement empirically validated cognitive-behavioral techniques for adult depression (see, e.g., Beck, 1995). Among these are the tracking of events that prompt negative thoughts and the listing of connections between these thoughts, feelings, and behaviors; thought stopping; thought substitution; and cultivation of more realistic appraisals of events and their potential impact.

Ecological contributors to depression must also be addressed. For example, Ms. Dern, the mother of 15-year-old Jim, experienced increased hopelessness and all-or-nothing thinking when Jim's urine tested positive for marijuana and alcohol. She told herself that things would never get better for Jim or for her, which made her feel hopeless, and contributed to her failure to implement consequences for drug use developed conjointly with the therapist. Ms. Dern's mother, who lived with her, often criticized her parenting, her low-paying job, and her appearance. Thus, before embarking upon cognitive strategies designed to combat all-or-nothing thinking (reinforced by her mother) and hopelessness, the therapist had to alter the interaction pattern between Ms. Dern and her mother that reinforced her negative thoughts and feelings, and to help Ms. Dern cultivate sources of social support. In this particular case, medication was not needed to help manage the symptoms of depression, which had really become problematic only since Ms. Dern's ailing mother moved in and Jim's drug use and threatening behavior began to escalate. In contrast, antidepression and antianxiety medications were needed to help manage the depression and social phobia of Michael's mother, Ms. Calhoun.

As discussed in Chapters 5 and 6, the MST team psychiatrist should be familiar with evidence-based guidelines regarding administration of pharmacological agents demonstrated to be effective for adults with specific disorders (e.g., Rush et al., 1998). The clinician, psychiatrist, and caregiver then work together to secure appropriate pharmacological care when it is needed.

## ANXIETY DISORDERS

For adults with anxiety disorders, pharmacological, cognitive-behavioral, and combined interventions may be warranted, depending upon the nature of the disorder. Cognitive-behavioral interventions often include structured relaxation training, exposure to anxiety-provoking stimuli, and monitoring of the linkages between events, thoughts, feelings, and behaviors described above.

When PTSD symptoms are demonstrated to interfere with a caregiver's ability to implement interventions effectively, the MST therapist should collaborate with the caregiver and psychiatrist to determine the most desirable course of action. A variety of treatment approaches for PTSD (cognitive-behavioral, pharmacological, psychodynamic, various types of group therapy) have been evaluated in studies with widely varying degrees of scientific rigor. Efforts to translate findings from these studies into treatment guidelines for practitioners have recently been undertaken; a volume edited by Edna Foa and her colleagues may be a useful resource for the MST team (see Foa, Keane, & Friedman, 2000). To summarize, the evidence is most compelling for the effectiveness of specific cognitive-behavioral approaches (exposure therapy, systematic desensitization, stress inoculation training, combinations of these, and cognitive processing therapy), while no data support the use of creative arts therapies. The evidence base for psychodynamic and supportive psychotherapies is very slim, and contraindications include the circumstances often faced by caregivers of youth referred for MST (e.g., life crises, low tolerance for additional anxiety and frustration).

Two caveats should be considered when consulting the volume compiled by Foa and colleagues and any other resource on evidence-based treatments. First, treatments for specific disorders (in this case, PTSD) are tested with individuals for whom that disorder is the primary referral problem. The impact on family members of the disorder and treatment is generally not examined, nor is the impact of the family context upon the symptoms of the disorder and their attenuation. Simply put, it is one thing to treat an individual self-referred for a study of a particular treatment, and quite another to treat that same adult when the primary referral problem is the imminent risk of placement of a youngster with serious emotional disturbance. Second, the treatment protocols tested in studies often involve specifically sequenced and structured sessions, treatment manuals, and supervision from an expert. Moreover, these treatments are usually not available in most communities. Thus, the MST therapist should be prepared to tailor techniques from empirically validated approaches to the unique strengths and needs of the caregiver and her or his context. Exposure therapy, for example, the most effective treatment for PTSD symptoms at this time, may not benefit individuals whose primary emotional response is anger rather than anxiety (Rothbaum, Meadows, Resick, & Foy, 2000). Moreover, anxiety and other symptoms often increase during the implementation of evidence-based treatments for PTSD (Foa et al., 2000). Thus, especially vigilant monitoring of the impact of these interventions on the caregiver's symptoms, family interactions, and progress toward ultimate treatment goals desired by the parent and family is necessary.

## SERIOUS AND PERSISTENT PSYCHIATRIC DISTURBANCES

Sometimes families referred for MST are affected by more serious disturbances of a caregiver or cohabiting relative that include psychotic features, such as severe depression or even schizophrenia. When the disorders are more severe, the MST team collaborates closely with the family member to determine whether the team psychiatrist should provide pharmacological treatment or an ecologically minded adult psychiatrist in the community should be consulted. In general, the responsibility for providing psychosocial aspects of treatment remains with the MST clinician, unless homicidal, suicidal, and floridly psychotic behavior on the part of the caregiver requires hospitalization or continued intensive community-based treatment from a team that includes a physician. Assertive community treatment (ACT; see Santos, 1996) teams of psychiatrists and nurses are available in many communities, and information about ACT and other empirically validated programs for adults with serious and persistent mental illness are catalogued by the National Alliance for the Mentally Ill. Such programs have been effective in reducing psychiatric crises and hospitalization. If a referral is made, however, the MST team remains responsible for understanding the nature of treatment being provided to the family member, assists the family in obtaining needed information from professionals treating the family member, and designs interventions and engages community resources that will increase the family's capacity to cope with what may turn out to be a chronic and difficult problem.

## Parental Substance Abuse

Parental substance abuse is targeted for intervention when it diminishes parenting capacity in ways that sustain the youth's behavior problems or present barriers to change. Alcohol and drug abuse are multidetermined and often co-occur with other psychiatric problems (e.g., anxiety, depression). Prior to designing interventions for caregiver substance abuse, clinicians must assess whether use or abuse is occurring, and whether that use or abuse is linked with referral problems, is a factor contributing to those problems, or is presenting barriers to treatment progress. Because the use of alcohol is normative in many segments of society and managed safely by many who use it, for example, one cannot assume that a caregiver that has once smelled of alcohol has a substance abuse problem. Functional indicators of substance abuse include unexplained missed days or poor performance at work; heightened marital or parent–child conflict; unexplained changes in the parent's availability at home; frequent private visits with previously unknown adults or the appearance of such adults in the home; changes in the parent's social circles; and unexplained changes (e.g., not due to recent unemployment, reductions in support checks, divorce, unusual medical or housing expenses) in the amount of money available to the family for food, clothing, and school. To determine whether such life problems are linked with substance abuse, the practitioner interviews the parent and family members and observes whether variations in the parent's behavior are associated with episodes of substance use or the aftereffects of such episodes. The physiological indicators of substance abuse vary in accordance with the substance in question (see Lowinson, Ruiz, Millman, & Langrod, 1997).

Treatment programs for substance abuse have proliferated in recent years, giving rise to clinical specialization (e.g., some states certify practitioners as substance abuse specialists) despite the absence of an adequate knowledge base regarding the effectiveness of various treatment models. No evidence supports the view that restrictive (e.g., hospital, residential) settings are safer or more effective than community-based treatments in decreasing drug or alcohol abuse in the short or long term (DHHS, 1999). For individuals with physical dependence on a substance, however, withdrawal may produce health risks that require medical management. Generic community-based psychotherapies such as supportive-expressive therapy, family therapy, group therapy, and interpersonal psychotherapy have yielded poor outcomes, whereas cognitive-behavioral strategies that include functional analyses of use and self-management planning show considerable promise (NIDA, 1999). The outpatient-based community reinforcement approach (CRA; Budney & Higgins, 1998; Higgins & Budney, 1993), which integrates contingency management procedures with interventions targeting changes in the client's ecology (family, vocational/educational, and social/recreational systems), have had the best outcomes with cocaine dependence and are used by several MST programs.

MST uses functional analyses and development of comprehensive self-management plans that address triggers for substance use in the social ecology. Such an approach is consistent with the focus of MST on assessing and addressing all factors that contribute to the fit of substance use. In addition to the usual MST focus on individual and ecological factors that contribute to a problematic behavior, the therapist and caregiver together identify in detail any thoughts, feelings, and behaviors leading to incidents in which the parent uses the substance. Behavioral (i.e., contingency management) and social-ecological interventions are used to address the factors supporting use, and cognitive-behavioral strategies are used to address thoughts that lead to feelings that increase the desire for the substance. Direct modifications of the adult's social circles are often necessary. The cultivation of friendships and activities involving nonusing individuals may be required. Limits might be set regarding the circumstances under which substance-using friends can be contacted. Monitoring of drug use via voluntary urine screens or breathalyzers may also be necessary, as intermittent sanctions of substance use tend to maintain abstinence. To effectively reduce substance abuse, sanctions should be implemented each time use occurs. Biological markers (e.g., urine, breath) provide reliable means to detect use. Other indices of substance use such as reports of family members and relatives, or charting of each hour or day in which use or nonuse occurs, should also be established. Contingencies are implemented in response to this information, and involve significant others. A spouse might promise dinner at a favorite restaurant in return for a week of nonuse. Points for nonuse might be earned and put toward the purchase price of a coveted item, and lost if use occurs. Or a family member might agree to accompany the parent to a new recreational or social activity.

## Practical Challenges and Basic Needs

Family members have great difficulty learning, growing, and changing when their primary physical, health, and safety needs are not being met (for a review, see Luthar, 1999). For example, parent–child affect and parental monitoring of child behavior may be difficult to improve when the caregiver works two jobs for an income that leaves the family at subsistence levels. When practical problems in living interfere with a caregiver's capacity to meet the child's needs, therapist strategies typically focus on helping the family to connect with people who can provide additional services and support.

Mr. Gordon, for example, was the divorced parent of two boys. No other caregiver had been involved in their upbringing for the past 5 years. The older son, William, was referred for MST following a psychiatric evaluation at the juvenile detention center. He was brought to the center following a schoolyard brawl in which he threatened to go home, get a gun, and shoot a fellow student. Mr. Gordon worked long hours for subsistence-level wages, and was unable to monitor William's whereabouts and too exhausted to cultivate positive affective interactions with him. Resolution of the immediate referral crisis required that Mr. Gordon take 2 days unpaid leave from work. The MST therapist worked with him to remove weapons from the home, meet with school officials and police about charges being pressed, and identify individuals who could monitor William's whereabouts when he returned to work. Initially, the MST staff were the primary sources of monitoring between the time William got home from school and Mr. Gordon got home from work. One neighbor and Mr. Gordon's brother were identified as possible sources of monitoring help, although the uncle's role had to be executed via random telephone checks because he drove a truck for a living and was often out of town. Next, the therapist worked with Mr. Gordon to find higher paying employment. In the interim, she helped him complete applications for subsidized school lunches and household heating. Until Mr. Gordon was able to change jobs, the therapist, uncle, and one teacher at school took the lead in helping William to get involved in a local economic development project that offered some compensation to inner-city youth who helped with a neighborhood clean-up effort. Once he changed jobs, and with continued monitoring help from his brother and neighbor, Mr. Gordon was less exhausted. William's pseudoemployment provided at least one topic for positive parent–child discussion, although the therapist had to provide coaching for these conversations initially. Additional interventions to enhance monitoring, discipline, and parent–child affective relations were needed, as were strategies to extend the social support available to Mr. Gordon, William, and his younger brother and to cultivate positive school–family linkages.

## Characteristics of the Child

Characteristics of a child such as a physical or developmental disability, chronic illness, ADHD, bipolar disorder, or difficult temperament may also contribute to difficulties in parent–child relations and ineffective parenting practices. Conversely, the nature of the parent–child relationship can either exacerbate or attenuate the difficulties inherent in a particular disability or temperamental predisposition. The therapist should understand the caregiver's perspective on the particular challenges associated with raising his or her child with special needs. In addition to tailoring parenting interventions to the problems observed in parent–child interactions, the therapist may need to help caregivers arrange for more frequent "breaks" from parenting than are needed by caregivers whose children do not have such problems. Examples of such breaks include having a weekend day away from home, visiting a relative without bringing the children, or having the child stay with a relative while the parent stays home. As described in subsequent chapters, such breaks may require the activation of informal or formal respite for the caregivers.

## Low Parenting Commitment or Affective Bond

For some parents, the process of developing and maintaining a strong affective bond with a child is challenged by the disability of the child or the parents. For other parents, the bond is established, but ruptured as a result of frequent and long-lasting parent–child separations that occur as a result of child placements outside of the home, changes in child custody arrangements, or the relocation, hospitalization, or imprisonment of a parent. Grandparents or other kin who are asked to assume the parenting role may love the child, but usually are not prepared for the ongoing monitoring, vigilance, and sacrifice the parenting role requires. They may well be committed kin, but not committed to the parenting role. Finally, for some parents, the demands of work, significant others, or other children erode commitment to parenting one or more children in the family.

Because many committed caregivers do voice frustration, a sense of helplessness, and a desire to place a child outside the home for treatment, therapists must be careful not to assume that lack of commitment is a barrier to treatment success without good evidence that this is the case. Occasionally, however, multisystemic strategies to change parent–child interactions are consistently met with half-hearted attempts, inadequate follow-through, or sheer lack of response from a caregiver. Usually one or more individual, concrete, or contextual factors described in this chapter account for such responses. Alternatively, the therapist may need to develop more effective engagement strategies or intervention strategies that address the caregiver's primary concerns. If, however, the team has ruled out individual, contextual, and therapist factors, commitment to parenting should be examined.

When evidence indicates that the primary barrier to treatment progress is commitment to parenting, the therapist's first task is to understand, from the perspective of the parent, how it makes sense that the parent has had a child, but now is ambivalent about continuing to care for that child. The information obtained from the parent often reveals beliefs and attitudes that can be changed. A parent may say, for example, that a live-in boyfriend, whom she hopes will help her care for the children, demands most of her attention and affection. The therapist can work with the parent and the boyfriend to establish reasonable boundaries around their adult relationship that do not compromise the mother's relationships with her children. Or a parent who travels a great deal for work may believe the income generated by the position is more important than his regular presence in the home. Alternatively, a parent may confess that he never intended to have children, and has periodically experienced deep ambivalence about parenting, particularly when the child's behavioral or emotional problems escalate. Appeals to the importance of the parent to the child's well-being may be helpful; the therapist should have evidence that the parent's periodic attention, praise, or otherwise positive attention is meaningful to the child when making such appeals. In any case, the therapist's job is to help change caregiver beliefs or attitudes that contribute to low commitment, and to identify what combination of changes would be required to persuade him or her to invest in the development of the child and in the MST treatment process.

In rare instances, intensive and extensive efforts to cultivate an adequate parent–child affective bond fail, and evidence indicates that the lack of such a bond precludes achievement of ultimate outcomes of treatment (e.g., physical safety of the child and others, effective management of depression, attendance and performance to capacity at school, etc.). The parent clearly and consistently indicates that he or she is unwilling or incapable of carrying out parental responsibilities, and the natural supports in the ecology of the parent and youth concur that their efforts to help the parent have not been effective. In such cases, the MST team works diligently to identify relatives or friends who would be willing to take on the responsibility of caring for the youth for the long term. In light of the fact that youngsters continue to love and feel loyalty toward parents, even those who have engaged in neglectful or abusive behavior, the youth is likely to have mixed feelings about becoming part of another family constellation. Moreover, changes in residence, school, and peer networks may occur as a result of the move. Thus, as with interventions for divorced and remarried families described below, the MST therapist must be prepared to help the youth and the new caregivers develop appropriate expectations regarding the new family constellation, to actively cultivate positive affective experiences, and to develop effective monitoring and discipline strategies. Therapists and caregivers must be respectful of the youth's attachment to the now-absent parent, yet vigilant against relaxing appropriate standards of behavior out of deference to the youth's recent experience of loss. Thus, for example, increased drug use is not an acceptable way for the youth to manage angry or hurt feelings about the estranged parent.

## INTERVENTIONS FOR RELATIONS AMONG COPARENTING ADULTS

Problems in the relationship between adult heads of the family often contribute to the referral behavior or constitute barriers to treatment progress. Interparental consistency in handling discipline is often compromised in the face of relationship problems, and conflict that is intense and unresolved can interfere with a parent's affective availability to the children and can contribute to aggressive or anxious behavior in children (Cummings & Davies, 1994). Research on marital therapies indicates that behavioral, cognitive-behavioral, and insight-oriented marital therapies are all more effective than no treatment in changing the behavior of spouses during treatment, but evidence regarding their longer term impact is mixed (Dunn & Schwebel, 1995). The intervention strategies described in this section draw upon several communications, cognitive-behavioral (perspective-taking, problem-solving) strategies used in these therapies.

Consistent with MST principles, marital interventions should target well-defined specific problems, be present-focused, address sequences within the marital dyad and between that dyad and other familial and extrafamilial systems, and require daily or weekly effort, including homework. The need to adhere to MST treatment principles is reiterated because practitioners new to MST and to marital therapy often revert to less structured supportive or insight-oriented approaches when the focus of intervention shifts from parent–child problems to marital difficulties. Common dilemmas reported by MST therapists are that practitioners have greater difficulty maintaining action orientation, directiveness, and consistency when intervening in marital, rather than parent–child, interactions.

### Setting the Stage for Marital Interventions

As with treatments for specific individual disorders discussed previously, marital therapies are tested with individuals for whom marital problems are the primary referral problem. Such is not the case for most families whose children are referred for MST. In light of the pressing nature of problems of youth with serious emotional disturbance, caregivers are typically focused on their child's problems rather than on possible marital difficulties. Thus, the MST therapist often must take special care to obtain an explicit agreement from the couple to address relationship problems in the context of MST. Sometimes neither, or only one, parent indicates that parental disagreements or marital problems are an issue. In such cases, the practitioner must be able to articulate incidents and sequences of behavior that link marital problems to the child behavior problems being targeted for treatment.

Having introduced the parents to the idea that marital problems may need to be resolved to attenuate behavior problems in their children, the practitioner sets the stage for conducting marital treatment in the context of MST. The therapist and couple need a shared understanding of the strengths and weaknesses in the affective and instrumental domains of the marriage before embarking upon interventions. It is often useful to begin discussion of the marriage with questions about what attracted the partners to one another initially, how they worked out decisions about who would take care of which household and family maintenance responsibilities, and what each expected in the way of emotional support, sexual compatibility, and so forth. Such a discussion serves at least three purposes: to identify strengths that can be used as levers for change; to "soften" the potentially angry stance each may have taken toward the other; and to reveal the extent to which conflicting assumptions about instrumental issues such as division of labor and affective issues such as emotional support or sexual relations may be unspoken. Couples often say that they had not actually worked out decisions, but fell into patterns almost unwittingly, or that the only time they talk about a particular issue is when they argue about it.

### Dealing with Negative Affect

Negative affect is easily generated and perpetuated in most couples with marital problems. The practitioner must help the couple interrupt the cycles of negativity that frequently occur in such marriages. Successful interruption of the behavioral sequences that constitute these cycles requires that partners learn and implement some basic skills. Consistent with cognitive-behavioral strategies for interpersonal problem solving, the following steps can help spouses to interrupt cycles of negativity. Each partner must:

1. Recognize that a negative behavior that is part of the cycle has been evidenced.
2. Inform the spouse that the negative behavior has occurred.
3. Explain the behavior and its corresponding meaning to the spouse in a nonattacking way.
4. Gain an understanding of the spouse's perspective regarding the negative behavior and the underlying circumstances that might have prompted the behavior.
5. Work out a mutually agreeable solution to the negative interaction.

Recognizing that a negative behavior has occurred requires that partners become aware of the precursors of conflict. Often, spouses will describe a sense of "here we go again" when they describe their feelings during the early stages of a conflict. The cues that signal "here we go again" can be used by the spouse to stop the sequence and reflect upon what exactly has set off the feeling of impending conflict. The therapist teaches partners to learn that the cues represent an "early warning system" for an imminent conflict. Taking a time-out when the warning occurs can help break the negative cycle. Immediately after the time-out, the couple comes back together to briefly explain their perceptions regarding the negativity in a nonattacking fashion. Explaining the nature of the perceived negativity is not the solution to the problem, but it can set the groundwork for a communication process that will help couples arrive at a satisfactory solution. When teaching couples to address their concerns in a more productive fashion, the practitioner will need to teach spouses to identify the cognitions each has in response to conflicts. When Ms. Lewis comes home from her day shift to a messy house, her automatic thought is, "If Marcus really cared about me, he wouldn't leave this place in such a mess," and this thought prompts hurt feelings. Mr. Lewis works extra shifts to earn more money for the family. When Ms. Lewis mentions the mess, his automatic thought is, "If Marge really appreciated what I'm doing for the family, she wouldn't bug me about the house," and this thought prompts angry feelings. Thus, the Lewis's argument about the messy house is actually fueled, in part, by beliefs that each partner does not really care sufficiently for the other and by the feelings that are linked with these beliefs.

A first step in interrupting this cycle is to help the partners identify the linkages between behaviors, thoughts, and feelings, both good and bad. A second step is to help each individual acknowledge the perspective of the other. Partners with marital problems often devote their energy to developing rationales for their own behavior rather than to understanding the mate's point of view. Shifting the pattern in which spouses do not listen to one another requires that each spouse use perspective-taking skills. Perspective taking requires that a person set aside his or her own view of a situation long enough to understand that another views the situation differently and the nature of that person's perspective. Again, in keeping with Principle 7 (interventions require daily or weekly effort), engaging couples in perspective taking usually requires the therapist to model the concept, provide multiple opportunities for practice within sessions, and assign homework that requires practice between sessions.

The next step in the problem-solving process is to work out a mutually acceptable solution. Doing so requires the cultivation of negotiation skills and the willingness to compromise. The practitioner must help spouses move from a mode of dealing with conflict that emphasized "winning" to a mode in which conflict situations are resolved in ways that allow both spouses to feel that they received as much as they gave. The priority is placed on each spouse doing whatever is reasonable to make the other comfortable with the outcome. The practitioner's responsibility is to help the couple develop a cognitive set in which each partner can say, "I believe I am right, but I understand my spouse's perspective too." When couples reach this level of cooperation, teaching them negotiation skills is fairly straightforward. When a couple has difficulty compromising, however, the practitioner may need to serve as an arbitrator. In the arbitrator role, the practitioner helps each partner identify concessions he or she is willing to make. The arbitrator role, unfortunately, does not promote the long-term maintenance of therapeutic change (Principle 9) because the spouses are not learning to resolve their issues by themselves.

## Changing Instrumental Relations

When marital conflict centers on instrumental issues such as household tasks, childcare responsibilities, and financial issues, the practitioner will often need to help spouses develop shared expectations regarding one another's roles. In doing so, the practitioner should help partners to develop the cognitive set that marriage is a 50–50 proposition that requires equal effort, time, and energy from each partner. While many couples will agree with this proposition, translating the concept into an equitable distribution of tasks often requires that one partner reconceptualize his or her ideas about the amount of effort he or she is required to devote to such tasks. Once reconceptualization has occurred, desired behavioral changes must be defined so that they can be observed and monitored (Principles 4 and 8). Examples include doing the dishes 3 nights a week (as opposed to just "doing the dishes"), picking the children up from school 5 days a week, and so on.

Spouses should be instructed to provide daily feedback to one another regarding their performance of instrumental tasks. Such feedback can occur at the end of the day, when they discuss their view of each other's efforts to change. Positive recognition is important, as such recognition can help break the cycles of negativity described earlier. Daily feedback also helps to put "bad" days in perspective, because couples have a more objective way of tracking how frequently bad days occur and can now place their occurrence in the context of "good" days. Spouses should also receive accurate negative feedback about their performance. One useful technique for providing feedback is to have spouses use a "report card" or "grade" approach. Throughout the feedback process, the practitioner must be continuously and accurately informed about the spouses' efforts (Principle 8). Such ongoing feedback will require the spouses to track one another's performance on paper, as is done when interventions designed to change the behavior of children are implemented.

## Marital Violence

Treatment outcome research in the area of marital violence is extremely limited, but suggests that even treatment approaches with short-term success (generally highly structured approaches involving meetings with both partners) do not prevent the use of physical violence in the long term (O'Leary, Heyman, & Neidig, 1999). Although the impact of conjoint versus gender-specific treatments on safety and effectiveness appears to be equivocal, marital adjustment is improved for men in conjoint treatments (O'Leary et al., 1999). Because most acts of physical violence occur during verbal arguments and involve mutual acts of physical aggression, therapist efforts to interrupt cycles of negative interaction, described earlier, can be helpful in preventing marital violence.

When physical abuse occurs repeatedly in a marriage, however, alterations in the usual approaches to marital treatment must be made. The MST therapist's first priority is to ensure that the abused spouse will be safe while undertaking marital therapy. Therapists should assess whether the abused spouse is fearful about participating in conjoint sessions. Based on studies of men in court-mandated abuse treatment (most of whom are divorced, separated, or single), a common concern in the field is that in-session comments will precipitate further abuse. Data from the limited studies of intact couples in which marital violence has occurred do not support this hypothesis, but such studies do not include couples in which a partner has been seriously injured (see O'Leary et al.,

1999). If a spouse fears reprisal for comments made in session, the therapist should not undertake conjoint sessions. Instead, referrals can be made to community-based, gender-specific treatment groups for women and for men. The women's groups typically include the development of safety plans and support networks and emphasize that the responsibility for the marital violence lies solely with the male perpetrator. Men's groups generally focus on taking responsibility for violent acts, and employ a variety of cognitive-behavioral strategies to identify cues to conflicts and physiological arousal and to enhance problem-solving skills.

As with all referrals to collateral services, the MST therapist and parent should examine the possible effects of those services (including safety plans) on the MST treatment plan and vice versa. Thus, for example, if a wife who attends groups generalizes, from the premise that physical violence is solely the husband's responsibility, to the premise that the arguments during which violence occurs are solely his responsibility, then therapist efforts to reduce marital conflict may be ineffective. If conjoint sessions are undertaken, it is not necessary that a partner acknowledge that a behavior constitutes abuse or that responsibility for abusive acts be accepted entirely by one or the other partner. However, both partners must be willing to focus on aggressive acts as a key problem to be solved.

### Divorced or Estranged Parents

Residential and nonresidential parents often have difficulties maintaining effective parenting practices following separation and divorce. When negative interactions between former spouses or the inability of former spouses to exercise interparental consistency contribute to a child's behavior problems, the practitioner's overarching goal is to enable the divorced spouses to act in the best interests of their children. Parents do not necessarily need to have an integrated, highly cooperative relationship to achieve the goal of redefining family relationships in a manner that will best promote children's well-being (Emery, 1999). Former spouses must, however, be able to make, keep, and renegotiate agreements about parenting tasks. Thus, the MST practitioner may have to help each parent devise acceptable means to communicate regarding such day-to-day issues as homework, doctor visits, birthday parties, and vacations. The practitioner should help the ex-spouses resolve conflicts that directly involve and affect their children. Such resolution often requires conducting a series of individual meetings with each parent prior to, and sometimes instead of, joint meetings. In addition, the practitioner may need to help the parent manage personal distress if that distress interferes with effective family functioning. Practitioners may find Dr.

Robert Emery's *Renegotiating Family Relationships* (1994) a useful adjunct to the MST manual when working with families engaged in ongoing conflict and custody battles that are contributing to a child's behavior problems.

In many cases, former spouses are able to coordinate discipline strategies, visitation schedules, and so forth with few difficulties. In other cases, however, normal parenting might be disrupted as parents grapple with changes in residence, income, and roles precipitated by the divorce. A parent may also attempt to appease the child and relax appropriate parental discipline out of guilt or concern about the divorce (Emery, 1994). Consequently, a coercive cycle of parent–child interaction can develop in which misbehavior that may have been punished previously is positively reinforced (e.g., appeasing the child), and parents are negatively reinforced for giving in to children's demands (i.e., parents experience relief from the child's negative behavior by giving in). As a result, children quickly learn the power of provoking parental guilt to achieve their aims. Rather than take up issues of child motivation in such cases, the MST practitioner should help the parent to consistently enforce rules of conduct and provide support as the parent builds confidence in his or her capacity to manage guilt-inducing and problem behavior. Divorced parents may also harbor concerns about the child's love or loyalty to him or her relative to the other parent. Such concerns sometimes present barriers to the parent's ability to exercise authority in the face of the child's comments comparing one parent with the other (e.g., "Dad doesn't make me do this"). For parents who have great difficulty "nonattending" to the content of the child's comments, the therapist might suggest that the parent focus on the behavior in question (e.g., the child won't clean up his room) rather than on the content of the child's comment (e.g., "Dad doesn't make me do this"). Although the child's comments may include realistic fears concerning conflict between parents, divided loyalties, and uncertainty about the future, such fears should be discussed at a later time, not during a parent–child interaction that revolves around limit setting, the completion of chores, and so on. Again, repeated practice, initially in the context of role plays, may be needed to help the parent remain steadfast in maintaining effective parenting practices following divorce.

## Stepfamily Adjustments

The multiple transitions experienced by children who experience divorce and remarriage can be disorienting even when they are well managed by all adults involved (newlywed spouses, former spouses, relatives). The four basic tasks facing stepfamilies are (1) creating a satisfying second marriage and separating it from the first; (2) integrating the stepparent into the child's life and vice versa; (3) managing multiple changes at the concrete, affective, and instrumental levels; and (4) developing workable rules for dealing with nonresidential parents and former spouses. Accomplishing these tasks is an ongoing process, with some evidence suggesting that it takes at least 2 years, and often longer, to establish new patterns that work relatively well for all family members (Visher & Visher, 1993). In many stepfamilies, bumps in the road to long-term positive adjustment are just that. For others, aspects of stepfamily functioning are so problematic that they contribute to behavioral and emotional problems in children. Factors that often contribute to these problems include unrealistic expectations about the stepfamily, conflicting parenting styles, premature or inappropriate delegation of disciplinary responsibility to a nonbiological parent, and marital problems.

UNREALISTIC EXPECTATIONS

Individuals often have unrealistic expectations about the family system, such as the expectation that the current family group is a re-created nuclear family. When the therapist has evidence that such expectations are contributing to a youngster's behavior problems, he or she may need to explain the developmental process of family reconstitution in terms that all family members can understand. The family may need to hear that developing an identity as a family takes time, that conscious effort is required to cultivate positive affective relationships and workable instrumental arrangements (e.g., who does which chores, how are money and time spent?), and that conflicts about preferred ways of doing things are normal. By reframing the thoughts and behaviors of parents and children as natural occurrences in the development of a reconstituted family system, the therapist can alter unrealistic expectations and foster a sense of cooperation among family members.

When stepsiblings are housed under one roof, conflicts about the manner in which resources, affection, and time are spent on the various children in the household often occur. If such conflicts appear to contribute directly or indirectly to a child's behavior problems, the practitioner should conduct a thorough assessment of the factors sustaining the real or perceived disparity. If real and significant disparities do exist that are not inappropriate to the developmental needs of children of different ages (e.g., infants should receive more parental attention than adolescents), the practitioner should address the basis of these disparities with the parents. On the other hand, if the disparities are more about perception than reality, such stepsibling conflicts should be normalized. Parents often expect that children from different nuclear families will develop positive affective bonds with one another simply because their parents love one another and they all live together. Although parents should develop and enforce rules for respectful behavior among all children in the household and should encourage activities that might stimulate positive affective experiences among stepsiblings, parents should not expect the children to experience or express positive affection for one another initially.

## Clarifying Parental Roles

When either lack of clarity regarding parental roles or inappropriate assignment of such roles contributes to the child's behavior problems, the practitioner should arrange to meet with the marital partners without the children present. The purpose of the meeting is to determine whether the spouses have, overtly or covertly, agreed upon the responsibilities each will have in caring for the biological children and stepchildren, how they came to this agreement, whether differences of opinion emerged, how such differences were handled, and so on. Such meetings often reveal that little time and attention have been devoted to the negotiation of parenting issues because the primary source of the spouses' concern was stabilizing the new marriage in the presence of the children. Alternatively, the newly married parents may have made an explicit agreement, but one that is likely to contribute to child behavior problems and/or family conflict.

Generally, stepparents are more successful if they first establish a positive affective relationship with a child, and follow the biological parent's lead in enforcing discipline strategies (Hetherington & Clingempeel, 1992). This sequence of parenting tasks (i.e., affective bonding first, guidance later) can be particularly difficult if the biological parent married, in part, to obtain help with parenting responsibilities. In such cases, the therapist should empathize with the biological parent regarding the many demands of single parenting, particularly when a child with serious behavior problems is involved. The therapist should also, however, dispel the myth that the stepparent can and should become the primary source of parental control in the household. To accomplish this goal, the practitioner will most likely need to teach the biological parent effective parenting strategies, create opportunities to practice those strategies that afford the parent success experiences, and solicit the stepparent's support for the biological parent. The biological parent's belief that the stepparent should be a disciplinarian is not likely to be dispelled unless the biological parent has been able to engage in effective parenting practices. The practitioner's task is to design and implement interventions that create such experiences.

## INCREASING SOCIAL SUPPORT
## AND CONCRETE RESOURCES

By virtue of the MST practitioner's frequent contact with multiple aspects of the family and neighborhood and community in which the family is embedded, she or he is in a strong position to assess the quantity and quality of social support available to family members. As indicated throughout this chapter, the availability of social support contributes to the well-being of caregivers and their children, and the lack of such support exacerbates conditions that compromise effective family functioning, such as depression, harsh or inconsistent discipline practices, inadequate parental monitoring, and so forth. The term *social support* actually encompasses four distinct experiences (Quick, Nelson, Matuszek, Whittington, & Quick, 1996; Unger & Wandersman, 1985). These are:

1. *Instrumental support,* such as helping to monitor a youngster after school, driving someone to an appointment, and financial assistance.
2. *Emotional support,* which include expressions of empathy, concern, love, trust, and caring.
3. *Appraisal support,* which provides affirmation or feedback, such as when Ms. Clarke's sister told her she was right to set limits for Rachel despite Rachel's tearful protests.
4. *Information support,* such as where to find the best prices on school supplies, or an auto shop that will take payment for repairs on an installment basis.

Rarely are all types of support provided by a single member of the support network. A parent may rely on several relatives to provide transportation to medical appointments, on a friend for moral support in troubled times, and on a neighbor for the latest word on clothing bargains for children. Across all these categories, most individuals rely first and foremost on indigenous, or naturally occurring, resources such as family members, relatives, friends, and colleagues.

### Assessing Social Support

To assess the nature and sources of support available to a family, therapists ask questions about individuals who might help the family in circumstances that reflect each type of support. For example, the therapist can ask, "Who makes you feel better when you're feeling down?" (emotional support); "If you couldn't get home from work on time, who could watch your children?" (instrumental support); and so on. The therapist should also assess how the family reciprocates the support received from each individual in the support system. Finally, individuals should be identified with whom contact stresses one or more family members. The same individual may provide support in some areas, but increase stress in others. Thus, a grandparent may be the source of important instrumental support, such as childcare, but also the source of depressive cognitions that compromise parenting skill, as was the case for Ms. Dern. Also, a source of support for one family member may be a source of stress for another. The girlfriend of a divorced father may be a source of emotional support to him and a source of stress to his daughter.

### Developing Social Supports

The nature and availability of indigenous social supports is multi-determined. Contextual factors that influence the quality and availability of social supports include neighborhood stability, transportation, social and cultural norms about social contact, language barriers, and availability of childcare. *Individual* factors can include health problems, psychiatric problems, substance abuse, cognitions (e.g., if I ask for help, they will think I am a bad parent), skills (e.g., how to ask for help and how to reciprocate), and resources such as time and energy, both of which can be in very short supply for parents who are trying to manage serious emotional disturbance in a youngster while raising other children and contributing to the financial support of a family. So, too, the *family* variables that compromise effective management of serious emotional disturbance (family conflict, marital discord, etc.) can interfere with the pursuit of effective social support. In addition, *neighborhood* factors such as high crime, rate of transience, and poverty; low levels of property ownership and employment; and poor transportation can present barriers to family linkages with safe and helpful community supports. Finally, *community* factors such as rural and urban configurations, economic base, and infrastructure (public transportation, parks, recreational and vocational programs) can contribute to the ease or difficulty with which instrumental supports can be cultivated.

As with the assessment and intervention approaches taken with individual caregiver- and family-level barriers to effective family functioning, therapists should identify the specific barriers to cultivation of social support that characterize a family and tailor intervention strategies accordingly. In the case of Jim and Ms. Dern, for example, several factors contributed to the social isolation that exacerbated Ms. Dern's depression, which, in turn, interfered with progress in managing Jim's substance use, irritability, and physically violent outbursts. First, the family lived in a subsidized housing development in a high-crime neighborhood, and Ms. Dern felt that she, her mother, and Jim were unsafe going out alone at any time. Second, to help make ends meet, Ms. Dern often worked overtime and 6 days a week at the nursing home where she was an aide, which allowed little time to cultivate social supports. Third, the family relied on public transportation. Fourth, Ms. Dern cooked special meals for her mother, who had experienced deterioration in eyesight and general health due to poorly managed diabetes, and tending to these dietary and health constraints further constricted time available for social contact outside the home. Finally, since Ms. Dern's mother had become her sole source of interaction outside of work, the mother's critical remarks exacerbated her sense of hopelessness and cultivated doubt that she would be of interest to others. As indicated in the discussion of individual factors that interfere with parenting practices, the therapist worked to change the negative interactions between Ms. Dern and her mother, and began to implement cognitive-behavioral interventions to address Ms. Dern's depressive cognitions. In addition, Ms. Dern identified another staff member at the nursing home who was a single parent, and the therapist and she devised a plan to schedule work breaks such that they could have coffee together at least once a week. They also identified a "Meals on Wheels" type of program that could accommodate her mother's dietary needs once a week, giving Ms. Dern one evening to spend an hour or two outside of the home after work. This change in routine had to be negotiated with her mother, of course; initially, the therapist coached Ms Dern through the interaction.

During the first week of the "night out" plan, Ms. Dern did not go out. Barriers to follow through included fear about walking the block from the bus stop to her apartment after dark, apprehension about being a stranger in a new situation, and not knowing whether public transportation would take her where she needed to go. Ms. Dern and the therapist determined that she could ask her coffee-break colleague at work what kinds of leisure activities she pursued, and contact the church she had stopped attending several years ago for information about possible church-related activities for adults. The colleague explained that she was dating someone, and that her limited opportunities for leisure usually involved him. She did invite Ms. Dern to join them on occasion, but Ms. Dern declined initially. Instead, she pursued the church option. Having called the church to ask for a list of activities and a membership roster, Ms. Dern identified a church acquaintance with whom she had lost contact. The two attended a local holiday craft show at the church; the acquaintance drove. In return, Ms. Dern invited the woman to have dinner with her and her mother on another evening. The Dern scenario illustrates that even the initiation of relatively minor changes to cultivate social supports can require attention to concrete (transportation), family (caring for grandmother), individual (apprehension about being a stranger), and extrafamilial (colleagues, church) factors.

Although MST interventions focus on developing sustainable, naturally occurring supports, many youngsters referred for MST have come to the attention of mental health, child protection, or juvenile justice agencies that have a legally mandated involvement with the child and family. Such agencies can provide resources such as transportation, subsidized childcare, components of an individualized education plan, or backup monitoring for a youth engaged in risky behavior (e.g., police or probation officer report a loitering teen to her parent, or help a parent find a runaway youth). On the other hand, the mandated involvement of agency personnel can be a source of stress, rather than support, for families. In addition, some agency procedures can present barriers to treatment progress for the MST team and family. Strategies for helping families to access formal resources for support and for effectively managing relations with agencies having mandated family involvement appear in the next chapter

## CONCLUSION

Because families take many forms and family functioning is influenced by both internal and external factors, MST family interventions subsume a variety of treatment targets. Although family interventions frequently focus on parenting practices, a constellation of interactions within the marriage (or its proxy), family, and social support system must often change to facilitate changes in parenting. In addition, individual risk and protective factors at the level of the child and caregivers must be considered in the development of family interventions. A caregiver who is clinically depressed cannot simply will herself to follow through with a behavior management plan. Thus, changing family interactions to support effective management of serious clinical problems in youth may also require the implementation of individual interventions for such problems as depression or substance abuse. The range of clinical competencies required to effectively execute family interventions across this multitude of bases can seem formidable; indeed, no single clinician is expected to possess all such competencies. With the ongoing training and support provided by the team and MST supervision process, however, clinicians and families together are often able to create and sustain change at multiple levels.

# CHAPTER 4

# Social System Interventions

## *Service System, School, and Peer*

MST gives explicit consideration and attention to the roles of extrafamilial systems in the development and maintenance of child and family difficulties. This chapter describes peer, school, and service system influences on youth behavior and provides guidelines for intervening when these influences are contributing to identified problems. In such cases, creating an effective family interface with extrafamilial systems is critical to achieving favorable outcomes.

## MST PRINCIPLES AND PROCESS APPLIED TO SERVICE SYSTEMS ASSESSMENT AND INTERVENTION

The MST principles and analytic process apply with equal force to clinicians' work with indigenous and service systems in the youth's social ecology. When evidence suggests that the behavior of key figures in the youth's indigenous ecology (e.g., family, peers, school, neighborhood, faith community) or service ecology (e.g., mental health, child protection, juvenile justice, courts) contributes to a referral problem or can enhance or encumber treatment progress, MST therapists assess the fit of the behavior. The same nine treatment principles, hypothesis testing, and accountability for outcomes MST therapists use in addressing family problems should be used to engage and influence external systems that have any bearing on those problems. For example, when faced with a social welfare caseworker's reluctance to allow a female youth to return home after a runaway incident, the MST team tries to understand the factors contributing to the caseworker's perspective. Such factors might include a judge's order regarding the disposition of runaway youths, inadequate engagement of the caseworker by the MST therapist, a history of negative interactions between the caseworker and the youth's caregivers, or the caseworker's beliefs about the causes of the clinical problems of the youth or her family members and their needed treatments. The therapist's task is to understand the concerns that drive the caseworker's reluctance, determine how the MST treatment plan addresses these concerns, cultivate caseworker "buy-in," and/or alter the plan to address the caseworker's legitimate concerns without compromising the ultimate goals of treatment. If, for example, the caseworker's reluctance is due primarily to the fact that the teen's uncle, her custodial parent, drinks alcohol regularly, the therapist would need to demonstrate either that the uncle's alcohol use is not a factor in the runaway risk or that other adults will monitor the youth's safety and whereabouts if the uncle has been drinking.

### Engagement

Therapists should take a *strength-focused approach* to working with all key figures in the youth's indigenous social ecology and relevant service ecology. Caregivers, teachers, caseworkers, probation officers, judges, and so forth are the experts at their jobs and should be respected as such. Schools, churches, and service agencies are organizations that have objectives to achieve, some of which are legally mandated. Formal policies and procedures provide a framework for the work done by their employees. Within this framework, individuals often develop preferred strategies for working that capitalize on their strengths. In addition, organizational climate and culture can influence children's service workers and child outcomes (Glisson & Hemmelgarn, 1998). Thus, the behavior of a particular psychiatrist, probation officer, or caseworker may be multidetermined by individual, organizational, and service system factors as well as by the behavior of the MST therapist and team.

To gain entrée into any system, MST therapists should *follow the established procedures* required for contacting employees, requesting information, requesting meetings, and so forth. For example, at some schools the principal must be notified before a therapist and caregiver can meet with teachers.

The therapist should meet with individuals in other organizations and systems *at times and places convenient for them*. Teachers are generally available before school starts or after the school day ends, but not during school hours. Probation officers may be most easily found between hearings at court. A caseworker overwhelmed with a high caseload may be reluctant to give up the relief of a lunch break to talk with the MST therapist, but could be willing to do so if the therapist buys the caseworker lunch in a pleasant setting.

When meeting with individuals outside the family system for the first time, the therapist should try to *understand the individual's perspective* on his or her role with respect to the referred youth and assess the individual's understanding of the MST treatment approach and the organization that houses the MST program. In general, the therapist should emphasize common goals, refrain from providing unsolicited advice, and take a one-down stance when asking individuals in another system or agency to work together on a particular intervention strategy. The latter point also implies that the therapist and MST team are clear about the specific types of collaboration they seek prior to requesting meetings or telephone time with colleagues. Just as meetings with family members should have specific objectives linked with intermediary and ultimate outcomes, so too should meetings with individuals in other systems. This rule of thumb does not imply that general informational meetings about treatment progress are prohibited; they should only be called, however, in response to stakeholders' need to have such information to continue productive collaboration toward the attainment of favorable outcomes. Of course, family permission to share such information must be obtained. Thus, if a referral agency requires updates prior to regularly scheduled hearings for youths with both juvenile justice and psychiatric involvement, the MST team would ensure that such updates are provided, pending approval from the family.

## Multisystem Interfaces

Just as the caseworker, psychiatrist in a hospital emergency room, and probation officer are embedded in organizations, these organizations are embedded in a larger service system. Thus, influences *within* and *between* organizations in the service system (e.g., the interface between mental health and juvenile justice) may influence the behavior of professionals in these systems. For example, "zero tolerance" policies established at some schools require teachers to report any youth who displays aggressive behavior to juvenile justice authorities. At the same time, the psychiatric hospital may not allow juvenile justice referrals access to emergency psychiatric evaluation and stabilization. Thus, a 14-year-old brought by a parent to a psychiatric emergency room following his assault on a teacher may be turned over to juvenile justice authorities rather than provided with crisis stabilization services. The therapist may need to work with the psychiatrist, hospital administration, police officer, and school to craft a solution that allows the youth to be evaluated and stabilized rather than released immediately to juvenile justice authorities.

One solution to the lack of coordination among child-serving agencies with different mandates is the system of care approach originally developed by the Child and Adolescent Service System Program at the National Institute of Mental Health (Day & Roberts, 1991) following guidelines described by Stroul and Friedman (1986). Although many communities have developed such systems of care, the extent to which a particular youth and family can benefit from the systems depends upon how well professionals in each service agency—including the one that employs the MST team—can work together with the family to ensure that effective treatment is provided. Thus, MST therapist or supervisor attendance at interagency service system meetings may help keep the relevant stakeholders aware of the MST program and contribute to general goodwill about collaboration. If the policies or practices of an agency attending the meeting can influence youth outcomes, direct contact with key players from the agency is needed to mediate these influences.

Attendance of the MST supervisor or administrator at interagency meetings can help promote mutual understanding about mandates and practices characteristic of these agencies and the MST program, but may not successfully avert problems that can be created at the level of the individual caseworker or therapist. For example, in one monthly interagency meeting, the family court representative described a new policy requiring drug screening and substance abuse treatment for any youth whose charges included possession of drugs. The nature of the required treatment was not specified. The MST supervisor attending the meeting informed the team of the policy change and suggested the clinicians wait to see whether and how the change would impact youths enrolled in the MST program. Shortly thereafter, a probation officer notified a family enrolled in MST that their daughter would be required to attend the local substance abuse agency's group-based adolescent treatment program as a condition of her probation. The youth had been arrested for possession and hospitalized for substance abuse treatment prior to referral for MST. Assessment of the fit of the probation officer's recommendation for treatment suggested that he had interpreted the family court policy as meaning referral to the local substance abuse agency was mandatory, when such was not the case. His recommendation also suggested that the MST therapist had not adequately engaged the probation officer in the MST plan for the youth's substance abuse problems. Because the supervisor had attended the interagency meetings, the MST team was aware of the court's policy shift, a change (i.e., treating antisocial youths together in groups) that was incompatible with the MST approach. The MST therapist was able to immediately address this concern with the probation officer. If the officer had not responded positively by withdrawing the request from the family, the MST supervisor or administrator would have met with the leadership at juvenile probation and the family court to effect the needed change in implementation of the policy.

## PROMOTING ACADEMIC AND SOCIAL COMPETENCE IN SCHOOL SETTINGS

### Assessing and Understanding School-Related Difficulties

Students with emotional and behavioral disorders often exhibit classroom behaviors that present obstacles to their social and academic development, such as noncompliance, aggression, disruption, and off-task behaviors (Wehby, Symons, & Shores, 1995). Moreover, poor school performance and behavioral and emotional problems in youth have mutually reinforcing effects; the former is a risk factor for the latter and vice versa (see McEvoy & Welker, 2001). Multiple aspects of the school context can exacerbate or attenuate problems that interfere with learning and positive social development. Among these are teacher–student and peer interactions in the classroom, peer interactions outside the classroom, classroom structure, school climate, administrative structure and leadership, community context, and linkages between family members and school personnel (for pertinent reviews, see Walker & Epstein, 2001). In addition, characteristics of the student and his or her family can impact academic and social performance at school. Thus, to understand the fit of a youngster's school difficulties, MST therapists should be prepared to obtain information and observational data about these factors.

MST therapists are responsible for engaging school personnel in the treatment effort, facilitating the development of effective collaboration between caregivers and school personnel, and designing interventions that are acceptable to caregivers and school personnel (and, as appropriate, to the child) and effective in reducing problem behaviors at school. The design of acceptable interventions generally requires that school personnel and caregivers share common goals regarding the youth's performance and behavior at school, and that the caregivers take the lead in intervention implementation. Teacher involvement in intervention design, implementation, and monitoring is equally important to intervention success, but must be sufficiently brief and straightforward to be easily integrated into the teacher's workload and classroom routines.

## TEACHER–STUDENT INTERACTIONS

Studies of classroom interactions suggest that students with emotional and behavioral problems receive teacher attention primarily for problem behaviors, low rates of positive praise or consequences for positive behaviors, and inconsistent responses to both positive and negative behaviors (Shores & Wehby, 1999). Teachers acknowledge that they feel poorly trained to handle disruptive behavior. The strategies teachers use to address problem behaviors in class are often more disciplinary and coercive than therapeutic (Walker et al., 1996). Interactions among students with behavioral and emotional problems and their teachers are often aversive to both. Unfortunately, the evidence base regarding promising school-based interventions contains only two reasonably rigorous studies involving youth with serious emotional disturbance (Hoagwood, 2000). Program evaluations of classroomwide or small-group social skills and self-management training programs have been conducted; however, these appear to have marginal effects with youth with behavioral and emotional problems (Quinn, Kavale, Mathur, Rutherford, & Forness, 1999). Thus, just as many caregivers of youth with serious emotional disturbance have tried multiple strategies to manage difficult behavior with no or limited success, so too have many teachers of such youth.

## PEER INTERACTIONS

As described in the final section of this chapter (on peer interventions), peer interactions are highly reinforcing of both positive and negative behaviors. Thus, classrooms or schools in which all youth have serious emotional disturbance present increased risks for "deviancy training" (Dishion et al., 1999) among peers. Conversely, research suggests that when educated in general education classrooms, students with emotional and behavioral disorders may gravitate toward peers with similar problems, but often also develop positive relationships with students who do not have disorders (Xie, Cairns, & Cairns, 1999). MST therapists should be prepared to work creatively and intensively with caregivers and teachers to maximize positive contact with prosocial classmates and to minimize association with problem peers in school. Because of the potential for deviancy training when youth are "tracked" into specialty classrooms or schools, a frequent goal of MST is to successfully transition youths from specialty classrooms to mainstream classrooms.

## SCHOOL ENVIRONMENT

The school is an organization, and, as such, has a mission (i.e., to educate all its children), administrative structure (e.g., principal, vice principal, etc.), operating policies, and an organizational climate that consists of attitudes, beliefs, and values about instructional practices, academic standards, behavioral norms, family involvement, and interfaces with other organizations in the community (Martin & Swartz, 1997; McEvoy & Welker, 2001). Any one or a combination of these factors can influence the experiences of students in- and outside of the classroom. Thus, the MST therapist's assessment of the fit of strengths and weaknesses in the school environment relative to a particular youth should be comprehensive and differentiated. For example, the team should be familiar with the major educational and disciplinary policies of schools attended by youth referred for MST. The threshold for student performance warranting evaluation for an Individualized Education Plan or for behavior warranting suspension may vary from school to school even within the same community. Moreover, implementation of evaluation or disciplinary policies may differ across grades, teachers, and individual children even within the same school. Similarly, the resources available to help teachers whose students have special needs may vary by grade, classroom, or teacher within schools. The physical infrastructure of the school and its location within the community can also influence the learning environment. Schools located in high crime areas may limit students' access to the playground or campus for safety reasons, whereas schools in other areas can make use of outdoor facilities with few safety concerns. In the latter scenario, extracurricular activities involving positive peers may be readily available on campus, while in the former the search for such activities may extend more quickly to community options beyond the school.

## FAMILY–SCHOOL LINKAGE

The quality of the family–school linkage is mutually determined by the reciprocal influences of family members and school personnel. Caregivers' involvement in their children's schooling is an important determinant of academic achievement and psychosocial functioning in school (Fine & Carlson, 1992). Key parental functions that support academic and social competence at school include monitoring school assignments, exam schedules, and grades; setting aside a block of time and quiet space for the child to study; supporting extracurricular school functions; implementing contingencies that are based on the child's efforts and performance; and providing overt support for the appropriate educational and behavioral demands and goals of the teacher. These functions do not require that caregivers themselves have a high level of education. They do require effective communication between school and home regarding assignments, extracurricular activities, and behaviors considered desirable and undesirable in the classroom or on school grounds. To this end, teachers and administrators must proactively enlist parental support for academic performance and social competence. Some strategies for enlisting support in the educational process are universal, such as sending home report cards or flyers about upcoming extracurricular events; others require individualization to a particular student, such as completing a daily checklist of student behaviors exhibited in class or scheduling brief parent–teacher telephone conversations at regular intervals. Therapists should assess how teachers, principals, and other key figures (e.g., coaches, school nurses, attendance staff) elicit family input, and the extent to which methods used are effective with the family of the youth referred for MST.

## SCHOOL–COMMUNITY LINKAGE

As the quality of education and school safety have become major issues on the national political agenda, how schools and communities develop collaborative partnerships has received increased attention (Trickett, 1997). Although MST therapists are not primarily responsible for forging partnerships between community institutions, they should be aware of opportunities and constraints that might influence collaboration between personnel at school and in other organizations when crafting interventions. For example, teachers and administrators disappointed with the school-based services provided by a local mental health center may not be receptive to the therapist's suggestion that the same agency provide a classroom "shadow" for a youth while she locates an individual in the natural ecology to perform that function. Alternatively, a school with formal ties to a community policing program may welcome increased visits from an officer to monitor suspected gang activity involving a youth referred for MST.

## FAMILY FUNCTIONING

As described in Chapter 3, various aspects of family functioning can influence youth behavior in multiple settings (at home, with peers, in school). Thus, therapists assessing the fit of school-related difficulties should understand the strengths and weaknesses in family functioning well enough to determine their impact on the child's behavior in school and on the family–school linkage. For example, family conflict that occurs at home before school begins can contribute to increased youth irritability and defiance at school later that day. Likewise, a caregiver with depression or substance abuse problems may be too tired to wake her children in time to catch the school bus. Alternatively, a child's difficulties at school may be a source of conflict at home. The therapist's task is to determine whether family difficulties are directly or indirectly contributing to identified problems at school.

INDIVIDUAL FACTORS

Finally, individual factors such as learning disabilities and low intelligence can interfere with academic performance and may contribute to disruptive behaviors in class. The disabilities, however, rarely lead to serious clinical problems by themselves. When a student is not achieving to reasonable expectations for her or his abilities, therapists and caregivers should be prepared to identify the contextual factors (at school, in the family, in the neighborhood, with peers) that contribute to the suboptimal performance, rather than assuming that the impact of identified disabilities or limitations cannot be altered. The therapist's role is to work with the child, family, teachers, and relevant specialists (e.g., learning disabilities expert, speech therapist) to design strategies that will enable the child to achieve to the level of his or her ability. Intelligence testing, achievement testing, and testing for learning disabilities are generally required to accurately identify a youth's intellectual strengths and weaknesses. The best validated test for intelligence testing is the Wechsler Intelligence Scale for Children–III (WISC-III; Wechsler, 1991). The best validated achievement tests for children are the Wide Range Achievement Test—Revised (WRAT-R; Jastak & Wilkinson, 1984) and the Peabody Individual Achievement Test (PIAT; Dunn & Markwardt, 1970). MST therapists should be familiar enough with the most commonly used instruments to determine whether the tests administered and their interpretation are appropriate to the task and understandable to caregivers. Dr. Jerome Sattler's (1992) book on intellectual assessment may be a useful reference in this regard.

## Implementing School-Related Interventions

ENGAGING SCHOOL PERSONNEL

As suggested in the first section of this chapter, engagement of school personnel requires MST therapists to respect the hierarchy and operating procedures of the school, meet with school personnel at times convenient for them, appreciate their perspectives and strengths, and understand contextual issues that affect these perspectives and their behavior (e.g., school policies, leadership, attitudes about performance, behavior). The therapist should not say or do anything to imply that the school is contributing to the child's problems; instead, the focus should be on the school as one important source of solutions to complex and multidetermined problems. As with all systemic interventions, the therapist should empathize with the experiences of stakeholders without falling into the trap of taking sides. Management of interactions among multiple players with differing perspectives, whether they are within the same system (e.g., embattled marital partners) or in different systems (e.g., teachers and caregivers) requires therapists to retain a broader social-ecological perspective and avoid being triangulated into one camp or another.

When the linkage between school and family is weak (e.g., school personnel and caregivers have had minimal contact) or embattled (e.g., communications have been primarily negative), therapists assess the fit of the linkage problems and design intervention strategies to build effective school–family collaboration. When the link is weak, school-related factors such as ineffective information-sharing strategies, teacher overload, or administrative problems may play a role. Ineffective information strategies can include Individualized Education Plan meetings in which school personnel use jargon that cannot be easily understood by caregivers, mailing educational testing reports with scant information regarding the meaning of those reports, and so forth. Alternatively, caregivers may not be aware of the importance of their involvement to their child's school performance or behavior or may feel intimidated by school personnel or uncertain about how to approach them. Such uncertainty or intimidation, may, in turn, be the result of negative educational experiences they or their other children have had. Therapists may need to coach caregivers through their uncertainty and intimidation, using role-played practice to prepare caregivers to approach school staff, and attending initial school meetings with caregivers. When jargon used by school personnel is difficult to decipher, therapists can teach caregivers in advance how to ask clarifying questions, and may model asking such questions themselves during the meeting.

When the school–family linkage is largely or entirely negative, commonly used intervention strategies involve coaching individual teachers and caregivers in how to engage in constructive communication and mediating meetings until such communication can occur. Steps in that coaching process often include helping teachers and caregivers to overcome negative attribution biases about one another or the child and refocusing their frustration about previous interactions on newly affirmed common goals.

When school disciplinary or educational policies contribute to contentious relations, therapists must also work with individuals who have
the authority to interpret, alter, and follow through with those policies.
The school principal, members of a school or district disciplinary board
or council, members of the school board, and judges are among these individuals. For example, a therapist would work with a principal and an
assistant principal to establish conditions under which a youth who is
repeatedly suspended for physically aggressive outbursts at school can
return to school before trying to build effective communication between
the teacher and the caregiver. Although the ultimate objective of MST is
to enable caregivers to successfully address systemic barriers to effective
collaboration, school-related crises with potentially long-lasting detrimental effects (e.g., a 15-year-old teen about to be permanently expelled)
are often occurring at the time a youth is referred for MST or shortly
thereafter. In such scenarios, the therapist and the family must balance
the goals of treatment generalization (e.g., preparing the caregiver to
manage systems barriers) against the expected outcomes of an imminent
action (e.g., permanent expulsion).

## ESTABLISHING COMMON GOALS

In general, the development and implementation of effective interventions for problems with school performance and behavior requires that
key school personnel and family members develop a shared understanding of the problems and possible solutions that are acceptable to all players. In some instances, such understanding is easily reached, and teachers
and caregivers have the resources, skills, and history of positive interactions needed to carry out intervention plans with relatively little assistance from the therapist. In other areas, the therapist must craft a mutual understanding of the problem and acceptable intervention steps.
Here, the therapist and the caregiver mutually determine the approach
to school personnel most likely to cultivate initial engagement and cooperation. Initial contact may involve the therapist–caregiver team; the
caregiver alone, with preparatory coaching by the therapist; or the therapist alone. Factors to consider when developing the opening strategy include caregiver preferences, the history of interactions between the
school and caregivers previous to MST intervention, indications of
school preferences for contact, and assessment of which participants are
most likely to engender the willingness of school personnel to collaborate. If a caregiver's frustration with previous school interactions is likely
to start a meeting on a contentious note, the therapist may suggest that
he or she meet initially with school personnel alone. Alternatively, a
teacher may indicate by phone that he would be happy to meet with a

caregiver, but also make disparaging remarks about that caregiver. In such a case, the therapist may suggest meeting with the teacher alone to get his perspective on the situation before meeting conjointly with the caregiver.

The purpose of initial meetings is to elicit the cooperation of key school personnel in the MST treatment process and to plant the seeds for family–school collaboration in that process. Therapist appeals to broadly construed common goals, such as facilitating the educational achievement of a youth and ameliorating problem behaviors that disrupt the classroom, are often helpful in this regard. Although the problems targeted for intervention are ultimately defined in more specific, focused, and objectively observable terms, broader goals can usually be agreed upon by teachers and caregivers alike. If teachers and caregivers have had contentious interactions in the past, the therapist may have to affirm for each party that the other views problem resolution as important, despite historically different perspectives on what those problems are or what their solutions might be.

## FAMILIES TAKE THE LEAD IN IMPLEMENTATION

The majority of the work for intervention implementation should fall upon the therapist and family. Many school-related interventions require caregivers to implement contingencies at home for the performance and behavior of the youth at school. The types of assistance required from teachers, administrators, coaches, or other school personnel generally take two forms: feedback to the therapist and caregiver regarding the nature and viability of interventions and assistance implementing interventions. Interventions that are complex and time-consuming are not likely to be implemented by teachers, most of whom are overworked, underpaid, and already grappling with the complex needs of many children when asked to devote individualized attention to one. For example, a short list of behaviors targeted for change may be developed conjointly by the teacher, caregiver, and therapist. The list might include arriving to class on time, listening without talking back when the teacher gives instructions, and raising a hand to ask for help rather than slamming books on the floor when frustrated with an assignment. The therapist would type the list and make copies to be checked off daily by the teacher. The caregiver, however, would be responsible for ensuring that the youth brings the list home, and would provide rewards and consequences based on the child's behavior at school that day. Similarly, although the teacher may be asked to list specific homework assignments on paper every day, the caregiver would structure the youth's time and space after school to facilitate the completion of homework, and would check to ensure that homework is completed before the youth goes to bed.

For all interventions, the responsibilities of the therapist, caregiver, teacher, and other key school personnel must be specified in detail. There should be no ambiguity regarding what each person does and how frequently. If, for example, a youth has the same teacher for two class periods, does the teacher check the list after each period or after both? Similarly, plans for monitoring the success of the intervention and the process for altering interventions must also be specific and clear. After how many days of partial success will the therapist and caregiver ask for a change in plans? Will the caregiver call the attendance office at 11:30 A.M. each day to see whether the daughter she dropped off at 7:45 A.M. has stayed in school? Or will the attendance staff notify the caregiver after the first skipped class? Such details must be revisited with all players each time an intervention is bootstrapped or when new interventions are introduced.

## PEER RELATIONS AND INTERVENTIONS

Peer interactions and friendships provide an important context for the development of emotional, social, and cognitive competencies. The development of positive peer relations and friendships is an ongoing and increasingly complex task that begins in infancy and continues through adolescence and early adulthood. In general, children and adolescents with positive peer relations are able to engage in perspective taking, empathy, collaboration in activities and tasks, and initiation and reciprocation of interactions across multiple social situations. Youngsters who have difficulty initiating or sustaining interaction and mutual give-and-take in relationships may be neglected (i.e., left alone) or actively rejected by their peers. Many of these youth do not develop serious problems. Conversely, many aggressive youths do have some prosocial friends or associates, while others associate primarily with peers who engage in antisocial behavior, who are not liked by prosocial peers, or who are both aggressive and socially rejected (for a brief review, see Farmer, Farmer, & Gut, 1999). Youths who are both aggressive and socially rejected are at highest risk for serious problem behaviors, including substance abuse. Moreover, just as positive interactions among youngsters are mutually reinforcing, so too interactions among peers with problem behaviors appear to be mutually reinforcing. Indeed, association with deviant peers consistently emerges as a direct and powerful predictor of adolescent antisocial behavior in multivariate longitudinal studies (see Henggeler, 1997b). Evidence suggests that even in treatment contexts directed by adults, such as counseling groups, youths with problem behaviors engage in mutual deviance training that exacerbates rather than ameliorates behavior problems (Dishion et al., 1999). Thus, a consistent focus of MST is to remove youths from deviant peer groups and to facilitate their engagement with prosocial peers.

## Family Processes and Peer Relations

Longitudinal research highlights the synergistic nature of the relationship between family and peer processes from infancy through adolescence (for reviews, see Parke et al., 1998; Pettit & Clawson, 1995). Caregivers influence their children's peer relationships in three major ways: (1) through the affective and instrumental qualities of caregiver–child interactions and childrearing practices; (2) as instructors or coaches regarding desirable behavior in social interactions (e.g., by suggesting that the child say hello or share a toy, or that an adolescent offer another youth a ride); and (3) as managers of their children's social lives who provide opportunities for social contact with children outside the family and manage the interactions of peers when supervising such contact. Parental influences in any of these capacities can be positive or negative. For example, parent–child conflict, frequent use of harsh and inconsistent discipline, poor monitoring, and low expression of affective bonding and involvement predict association with negative peers (Patterson, 1997). Conversely, effective monitoring and discipline strategies and high levels of family support and involvement can buffer the effects of youth involvement with deviant peers and protect against association with drug-using peers (Hawkins, Catalano, & Miller, 1992). Similar patterns of association between parental discipline, support, and monitoring and peer relationships emerge for a wide array of high-risk and problem behaviors in youth (Ary, Duncan, Duncan, & Hops, 1999). Finally, despite adolescents' developmentally appropriate increases in peer, versus family, activities, caregivers remain important sources of guidance, emotional support, values orientation, and instrumental help with respect to issues such as education, jobs, and planning for the future (Parke et al., 1998).

## Assessing Peer Relations

### SOURCES AND TYPES OF INFORMATION GATHERED

The primary purpose of assessing the youth's peer relations is to enable the MST therapist and family to identify characteristics of those relations that contribute to behavioral and emotional problems and that can be used to attenuate such problems. To obtain a comprehensive picture of the strengths and weaknesses in the youth's peer interactions, the therapist gathers information from direct observations of the youth in a variety of contexts involving peers and from interviews with family members, teachers, and the youth. Observations of interactions with peers should occur at home, in school (e.g., in class, at lunch, on school grounds), in the neighborhood, and at other sites at which the youth participates in organized or casual activities with other same-aged, older, and younger peers. Information about the youth's peer relations should also be obtained from the youth's caregivers, parents of the youth's peers, teachers, coaches, and neighbors who know the youth and family. Likewise, fairly mundane practical activities can provide the caregiver with regular opportunities to observe and/or manage peer interactions. For example, a parent can ride the subway to her daughter's basketball game with other team members, meet a son at the bus stop, or invite new acquaintances to the home (and require such visits) before letting a son or daughter go out with them. The purpose of gathering these data is to enable the therapist and family to assess dimensions of the youth's peer relations that may contribute to or prevent further emotional and behavioral difficulties. These dimensions include:

1. Number and nature of acquaintanceships versus friendships.
2. Reputations of acquaintances and friends.
3. Social functioning of acquaintances and friends.
4. Intellectual functioning of acquaintances and friends.
5. Homogeneity versus heterogeneity of peer group (e.g., all deviant or rejected peers; some antisocial, some prosocial peers). If the youth's peer interactions involve some positive and some negative peers, what are the settings and activities in which the adolescent associates with the deviant versus the prosocial peers, associates with others, or begins to withdraw?
6. Sociometric status of the youth (well liked, disliked, leader, loner, neglected, or actively rejected) and behaviors that appear to contribute to that status (e.g., is aggressive or withdrawn vs. is appropriately assertive but not aggressive, doesn't withdraw when uncomfortable in social situations).
7. Family–peer linkage. Do the caregivers know the youth's peers and peer activities? Do they express interest in the youth's activities?

## Peer Interventions

### CHANGING PEER AFFILIATIONS

When the therapist and family find that association with deviant peers contributes to a pattern of problem behavior (e.g., truancy, runaway behavior, substance abuse, fighting, noncompliance with medications needed to effectively manage depression or ADHD, etc.), interventions aimed at reducing the youth's affiliation with deviant peers and increasing his or her affiliation with prosocial peers are necessary. Such interventions rely upon the therapist to help caregivers to:

- Monitor the youth's whereabouts.
- Increase parental contact with the youth's peers and parents of peers.
- Implement very unpleasant consequences when the youth contacts antisocial peers and positive consequences when the youth contacts positive peers.
- Facilitate the youth's participation in prosocial activities such as sports teams, church groups, recreation center activities, and afterschool volunteer or paid employment.
- Help the youth identify areas of competence and interest.

The details of the intervention strategies vary in accordance with the strengths of the particular youth, family, school, neighborhood, school, and community. In addition, interventions may vary as a function of the extent and intensity of the youth's association with peers with problem behaviors. Many youth referred for MST have friendships with a mixture of peers with and without serious problems, while others affiliate only with problem peers.

## CAREGIVERS AS KEYS TO PEER INTERVENTIONS

Consistent with MST Principle 9, interventions to address problematic peer relations must be sustainable in the absence of the MST therapist. Thus, caregivers are key agents of change in the realm of peer relations. Caregivers are, or should become, sources of monitoring and discipline strategies needed to reduce opportunities to affiliate with problem peers; experts in the interests and talents of their sons and daughters, even if these have been eclipsed by emotional or behavior problems; facilitators of exposure to community activities in which prosocial peers can be found; and liaisons with the parents of prosocial peers and the adult supervisors of these activities.

## PREPARING CAREGIVERS TO INTERVENE

Caregivers' efforts to remove a son or daughter from a deviant peer group or to prohibit contact with a particular peer are usually hotly contested by the youth. Thus, the therapist–caregiver team should follow several guidelines when attempting such interventions.

1. Help the youth see the disadvantages of associating with problem peers without berating, belittling, or insulting peers who are valued by the youth. To follow this guideline, caregivers will need concrete evidence that association with questionable peers is linked with negative consequences for the youth. Therapists should be prepared to help caregivers collect such evidence. For example, the fact that a mother dislikes the way a peer dresses does not constitute evidence that the peer negatively influences her daughter, whereas the fact that the peer and daughter are often together when the daughter skips school does.

2. Peer validation is powerful; even among groups of peers who engage in negative behavior individuals typically feel important and valued. Thus, caregivers may have to acknowledge that the youth has positive feelings about the deviant peers while focusing on the consequences in the youth's life of affiliating with a deviant peer or peer group. The feelings the youth has about his or her peers should not be debated. Accepting the reality that the youth has positive feelings despite the fact that the caregiver typically does not, the task is to cultivate a shared parent–child understanding of what constitutes a sufficiently negative consequence to render prohibition from the peers necessary. Developing a shared understanding of negative consequences is often easier if arrests, police involvement, or placement outside of the home have occurred as a consequence of affiliation with deviant peers. Absent such events, therapists should be prepared to work with caregivers to identify goals or desires of the youth that are likely to be thwarted by continued affiliation with deviant peers. For example, dropping out of school may be acceptable to a 16-year-old girl whose 18-year-old boyfriend and his buddies did the same, but completely unacceptable to a caregiver. The caregiver might talk with the daughter about the wages she can expect to earn without a high school degree, and how long it will take to earn the money needed to purchase the car, apartment, and clothing she expects to own in short order.

3. Therapists must prepare caregivers for battle. Caregivers must have the instrumental, emotional, appraisal, and informational support (see Chapter 3) of family members, friends, coworkers, and the parents of peers prior to implementing interventions designed to minimize their child's contact with valued but deviant peers and increase his or her contact with unfamiliar but prosocial peers. Even when such support is forthcoming, the therapist should be prepared to provide substantial support initially—for example, by taking phone calls at midnight when the youth doesn't return home, arriving on the scene when the youth

does return and the caregivers try to implement a harsh consequence, and so forth. If, as occasionally happens, peer interventions require such extreme measures as tracking a youth's whereabouts when he or she is with deviant peers who may temporarily house or hide the youth, the caregivers may also need to enlist the support of more formal community supports such as probation officers, community police, and social service staff.

## OVERCOMING PEER NEGLECT OR REJECTION

When a youngster is socially isolated, actively rejected, or neglected (left alone) by same-aged peers, the therapist and family should assess which aspects of the youth's interpersonal behavior may be contributing to the lack of peer bonding and/or social isolation. If impulsive or aggressive behaviors are primary contributors to disrupted peer relationships, the therapist should make sure that family and family–school interventions are addressing all the factors that sustain these behaviors and that biologically influenced contributing factors, such as ADHD, are carefully assessed and managed. In some cases, cognitive deficiencies and distortions contribute to inept or aggressive peer interactions.

If aggression or impulsive behavior do not appear to be primary obstacles to the development of peer relationships, the therapist should work with the youth and family to identify which of several areas of interaction known to be associated with successful peer relations may be problematic for the youth. In general, youth who experience social rejection or neglect often withdraw from social situations, have difficulty initiating and sustaining positive give-and-take in conversations and/or activities, and act in ways that are not socially acceptable and valued by same-aged peers. Withdrawal and failed efforts at maintaining positive social give-and-take often result in peer avoidance, which, in turn, minimizes the positive peer contact necessary for the unskilled adolescent to learn alternative prosocial behaviors. Moreover, physical attractiveness, hygiene, and conformity with peer norms for dress and appearance can influence acceptance among peers, though research indicates that these factors are not as central as behavioral, cognitive, and emotional competencies to the development of positive peer and friendship relations.

## FAMILY INVOLVEMENT IN INTERVENTIONS

To increase the likelihood that learned skills generalize to home and neighborhood settings, every effort should be made to include caregivers in interventions to improve the social interaction skills of youth who are isolated, neglected, or rejected by peers. As with all MST interventions, the therapist should be aware of patterns of family interaction that may be contributing to the youth's problems interacting with peers. For example, the family itself may be socially isolated. One or both caregivers may be socially anxious or relatively unskilled in social interactions. Caregivers may not be aware of the important role they play in arranging opportunities for their children to engage in social interaction (e.g., by seeking out community activities, allowing peers to visit, providing rides to the mall). Thus, prior to and while implementing individualized cognitive-behavioral and social skills training techniques, the MST therapist should implement intervention strategies to address the specific factors believed to contribute to the peer problems. Presumably, for example, interventions to reduce verbal and physical conflict between family members would be in place, and the therapist would be working with caregivers to identify and access activities in the community that provide peer contact.

## PEER INTERACTION INTERVENTIONS

When evidence indicates that a youth's cognitive distortions or deficiencies contribute to his or her problematic interactions with peers, cognitive-behavioral interventions targeting the youth's perception of social interactions and his or her responses may be required. For example, a youth who perceives a classmate's dispassionate glance as pity and responds with irritation and withdrawal would be instructed by the therapist to consider alternative reasons for the glance (e.g., the classmate notices the youth's new shoes or is curious about why the youth missed class for a few days). Then the therapist and youth would practice befitting behavioral responses. The therapist would also coach caregivers to help the youth interpret social events more accurately, and help them establish rewards and consequences for appropriate and inappropriate behavioral responses. To conduct such interventions the caregivers must be aware of the times and places in which the youth has opportunities to engage others, and must have access to reports of the nature of peer interactions. Teachers, neighbors, adults in charge of activities for youth (e.g., church groups, sports teams, music groups), and kin can be helpful observers in this process. Once attribution biases and alternative interpretations of social behavior have been identified, the problem-solving steps outlined below are undertaken to ensure that the youth has a range of appropriate responses to the kinds of situations that place him or her at risk for ineffective (anxious, depressive, or aggressive) responses.

SOCIAL PROBLEM-SOLVING SKILLS INTERVENTIONS

Universal social skills training programs are often implemented with youth identified as having emotional and behavioral disorders (Quinn et al., 1999). These programs identify critical social skills to be improved; explain, demonstrate, and model these skills; provide opportunities for youngsters to practice with coaching; and identify situations in which the new skills should be practiced. The impact of such training appears to be minimal (Quinn et al., 1999), however, possibly because many youths with serious emotional disturbance do not have social skills deficits and the interventions are not individualized to the specific circumstances facing a particular youth at home, at school, or in the neighborhood. By virtue of their familiarity with all aspects of the youth's social ecology, MST therapists are in a unique position to help overcome these barriers to social skill intervention success.

Social skill is not a unitary concept. It includes acquaintanceship skills (the initiation of friendships and peer interactions); communication skills, such as asking questions to initiate a conversation, appropriate self-disclosing to promote closeness, and making suggestions and invitations; sharing and cooperation skills; and problem-solving and conflict resolution skills (Bierman & Montminy, 1993). Thus, therapists should be careful to assess which types of skills are lacking, and then tailor interventions accordingly. Steps central to problem-solving and conflict resolution strategies tested in treatment studies include:

- Identifying the problem in dispassionate terms ("We both want to sit next to Jim on the bus" not, "Max is a jerk for not letting me sit in my seat on the bus").
- Understanding that there are multiple perspectives on the problem (Max saw the open seat and wanted to sit next to James).
- Generating all possible solutions (shove Max off the seat, ask Max to move, take a different seat today and ask to sit next to Jim tomorrow).
- Evaluating the positive and negative consequences of the solutions (get suspended for shoving Max; inconvenience Max, possibly making him angry; miss out on sitting next to Jim this time, but sit next to him tomorrow).
- Selecting solutions that capitalize on positive consequences and minimize negative consequences (miss out on sitting next to Jim today, and sit next to him tomorrow).
- Practicing the implementation of the solution (with the therapist and a parent or responsible family member initially).

To facilitate social competence with respect to problem-solving or any of the other skills needed to establish and maintain friendships (e.g., making introductions, asking appropriate questions, making appropriate disclosures), the therapist and caregiver conjointly provide instruction in the particular skill to be learned, model the behavior, provide opportunities for the youngster to practice, and provide verbal reinforcement and corrective feedback after observing the practice. The interventions should be explained to caregivers so that they can reinforce the newly developing skills and become involved in coaching the youth in the absence of the therapist.

## CONCLUSION

The guidelines for engagement, assessment, and intervention with extrafamilial systems are equally applicable to the MST therapist's work with formal systems (e.g., schools, courts, agencies) and indigenous systems such as the peer group of a referred youth. To gain access and to cultivate initial engagement, the MST therapist follows established organizational procedures. The therapist schedules calls, meetings times, and locations convenient for the individuals (e.g., parents of peers, teachers, judges, caseworkers). The therapist obtains the individual's perspective on his or her role with the referred youth and family, and emphasizes goals shared by the individual and the agency he or she represents, the family, and the MST team. Intervention strategies involving extrafamilial systems should be clear, closely monitored, and bootstrapped in accordance with ongoing assessment of the success or failure of the intervention and, in the latter case, of barriers to intervention success. Such barriers may occur at the level of the individual, the organization (e.g., agency, school) within which the individual is embedded, or the interfaces between multiple systems.

# PART II

# Adapting MST to Treat Youths with Serious Emotional Disturbance

MST programs have traditionally focused on juvenile offenders at imminent risk of placement due to their serious antisocial behavior. Although a substantive percentage of these offenders had relevant psychiatric comorbidities, MST treatment emphasized attenuating the antisocial behavior that was leading juvenile justice authorities to recommend placement in a secure setting to protect the community. As such, MST treatment addressed key risk factors by, for example, promoting parental competency to monitor and supervise their son or daughter and disengaging youths from deviant peer groups. To implement such interventions, therapists primarily required skill in changing interpersonal relations and addressing system-level influences on outcomes. Psychiatric involvement was rarely needed because mental health emergencies (e.g., suicidal behavior) and pharmacological interventions were infrequent. When youths presented with mental health emergencies (e.g., suicidal ideation) or were in need of pharmacological intervention (e.g., ADHD), team members consulted with physicians in the community.

As MST was implemented for youths presenting psychiatric crises (i.e., suicidal, homicidal, psychotic) within the context of an NIMH-funded randomized clinical trial, however, significant adaptations in the MST service delivery system were required to ensure the safety of the youth and the community (Henggeler, Rowland, et al., 1997). These adaptations included the allocation of more intensive clinical resources, close involvement of psychiatry specialists, specification of crisis stabilization protocols, and the development of short-term placement options that would facilitate the MST treatment process. The following three chapters detail the adaptations of MST needed to treat youths with serious emotional disturbance who are referred from the mental health system.

# CHAPTER 5

# Addressing Psychiatric Emergencies

*Staffing, Assessment, and Intervention Protocols*

with SUSAN G. PICKREL

---

This chapter describes staffing patterns, assessment strategies, and intervention protocols to stabilize psychiatric emergencies, including suicidal, homicidal, and psychotic behavior. Emphasis is placed on maintaining youth, family, and community safety while stabilizing the crisis outside the hospital setting, if at all possible. Successful implementation of these protocols is a first step in resolving the problems that precipitated the crisis.

---

## GOALS OF MST CRISIS INTERVENTION

MST crisis intervention is conceptualized as a therapeutic alternative to the immediate out-of-home placement (e.g., psychiatric hospitalization, residential treatment, detention) of youth with serious emotional disturbance presenting acute psychiatric emergencies. *Crises* are defined as

---

Susan G. Pickrel, MPH, MD, Medical Director of Child and Adolescent Psychiatry, Mercy Medical Center, Roseburg, Oregon.

(1) the youth is acutely and imminently at risk of harm to self or others (e.g., homicidal, suicidal, psychotic), or (2) the youth's needs far exceed the functional capacity of the immediate social environment, and consequently place the youth at risk of out-of-home placement. The goals of MST crisis intervention are to (1) ensure client safety, (2) provide emergency services in the natural environment, (3) prevent unnecessary out-of-home placements, (4) empower caregivers to deal effectively with current and future crises, and (5) reduce the length of the stay in out-of-home placements when they occur.

## MST CRISIS TEAM

The main purpose of the crisis team is to help stabilize acute situations involving clients at risk of harm to themselves or others. Each crisis team member has specific duties and shares responsibility in designing and implementing crisis plans that best meet the needs of the client and family. Crisis teams are extensions of MST treatment teams and include an administrator, an MST supervisor, therapists, crisis caseworkers, and child psychiatrists. A brief overview follows of the roles each crisis team member plays in crisis planning and intervention. All personnel must develop a thorough understanding of existing federal and state ethical guidelines and laws concerning situations that may occur in crisis treatment (e.g., therapeutic holds, commitments, reporting abuse or neglect). They should also be familiar with the organizational and procedural regulations (e.g., agency mission, culture, administrative structure) of relevant collateral agencies (e.g., juvenile or family court, probate court, social service agencies).

### Administrator

This master's- or doctoral-level person has overall responsibility for the MST program and coordinates both administrative and clinical aspects of the crisis team. Clinically, the administrator's primary role is developing formal supports from community agencies for various aspects of the MST program, including current and future crisis treatment planning. *Formal support* refers to agencies or entities that provide resources or services (e.g., schools, social service agencies). Toward this end, the MST administrator meets formally and informally with representatives from various organizations in the community most likely to be involved in MST crisis treatment plans. These agencies include the local police, emergency rooms, social services, temporary shelters, resident advisors (from housing developments within the program's geographic area), mobile crisis services, and runaway shelters. In addition, the administrator ensures that crisis plans, as developed by the treatment team, are consistent with MST conceptualizations of behavior and within the financial constraints of the organization.

## Supervisor

This master's- or doctoral-level individual is primarily responsible for supervising MST therapists and ensuring treatment fidelity. MST supervisors help clinicians acquire and implement the conceptual and behavioral skills required to deliver MST (Henggeler & Schoenwald, 1998). The supervisor's two primary responsibilities as a member of the crisis team are *client safety* and *ensuring that crisis plans are consistent with MST conceptualizations of behavior*. Thus, the MST supervisor engages in four tasks.

1. The supervisor oversees the development of a crisis plan that (a) ensures the safety of the client, family, and community; (b) is informed by MST treatment principles; and (c) is based on the strengths and needs of the targeted youth and family.

2. The supervisor communicates the roles and expectations of the crisis plan to all concerned. Generally, the supervisor communicates the crisis plan to the members of the treatment team (e.g., MST administrator, therapists, psychiatrists, crisis caseworkers, other team members) and collateral agencies involved with the case or likely needed to carry out the crisis plan (e.g., police, crisis shelter). To the treatment team, the MST supervisor communicates the following information: (a) the specifics of the plan and its conceptual rationale and relevance to overarching treatment goals, (b) parameters of interactions with caregiver and youth (i.e., how to work with the youth and family informed by previous interactions with them), and (c) therapeutic tactics (e.g., behavioral contingencies). The MST supervisor, in conjunction with the MST administrator, also communicates relevant aspects of the crisis plan to collateral community agencies or significant others (with signed releases). For example, some crisis plans call for police or crisis shelter personnel to respond to clinical exigencies and meet specific clinical needs (e.g., safety checks, visual observation). Thus, the MST supervisor or administrator must procure support prior to implementation of the safety plan from the police or shelter administrator and communicate the exact help requested.

3. In conjunction with the MST administrator, the supervisor engages in activities designed to develop and maintain collaborative relationships with collateral community agencies. This role is crucial in both

developing and implementing crisis plans that are dependent upon services provided by collateral agencies (e.g., police, social services, shelters, etc.).

4. The MST supervisor facilitates the team's interface with the child psychiatrists to ensure that consultation occurs when indicated.

## Therapist

This master's-level individual has primary responsibility for developing crisis plans informed by MST treatment principles and the family's strengths and needs. The MST therapist should have experience using behavioral interventions (e.g., contingency procedures, skills training, problem solving, cognitive restructuring) and family therapy. The therapist must be well versed in MST and be able to apply multisystemic principles when working with youth with serious emotional disturbance and their families.

## Crisis Caseworker

This bachelor's-level individual is a critical member of the crisis team. The crisis caseworker responds to emergencies, implements crisis plans, and gathers important information on the psychosocial functioning of the youth and family and any contextual factors affecting such functioning during a crisis. Crisis caseworkers' responsibilities are grouped into two categories: ancillary activities and crisis management.

### ANCILLARY ACTIVITIES

One responsibility of the crisis caseworker is providing "ancillary" services to the treatment team. Ancillary services are conceptualized as treatment team and therapist "support" and are designed to free time for the clinical activities of other team members. Ancillary services may include clinical (e.g., client transportation, client monitoring) and administrative (e.g., making phone calls, scheduling appointments, gathering information about resources and completing paperwork) tasks.

### CRISIS MANAGEMENT

The most important responsibility of the crisis caseworker is crisis management. Crisis management entails many activities best categorized by function. These functions include crisis assessment, crisis plan development and implementation, communication, and resource procurement.

A more detailed discussion of these functions appears in subsequent sections.

## Child Psychiatrist

The child psychiatrist's (or team of psychiatrists') overall responsibility is medical coverage for the crisis team. The MST child psychiatrist provides the following services: 24-hour/7-day-per-week medical coverage; psychiatric evaluations for youths and family members; clinical consultation with MST treatment teams; community liaison with outside physicians/psychiatrists concerning medical or psychiatric care of youth, caregivers, and family members; and emergency psychiatric evaluations (e.g., in the community, emergency room, shelter). In addition, the child psychiatrist coordinates psychopharmacological interventions and evaluations. To maintain adequate familiarity with clinical cases and to stay abreast of the psychiatric needs of clients and family members served by the treatment team, the child psychiatrist attends staff meetings and maintains frequent contact with the MST supervisor. The psychiatrist works with the supervisor to ensure that team protocols for therapeutic holds, commitments, and charting meet local and professional standards of care.

In summary, MST crisis team members have general and specific responsibilities during psychiatric emergencies. Consistent with the philosophical underpinnings of MST, however, each member of the treatment team is accountable for client outcome. That is, crisis team members share responsibility for crisis plan development and implementation.

## CRISIS TEAM INTEGRATION

This section focuses on integrating the various crisis team responsibilities, specifically how crisis team members work together and make decisions during psychiatric emergencies (see Figures 5.1 and 5.2). The crises encountered can be placed in one of two categories: predictable and unpredictable. A *predictable crisis* is clinically anticipated and precipitated by an intervention or set of contextual factors. For example, behavioral interventions such as extinction-based procedures (withdrawal of reinforcement) in the beginning of an intervention temporarily increase the frequency, intensity, and strength (i.e., extinction bursts) of the behavior one is trying to decrease. Also, the crisis assessment may reveal that cer-

tain contextual factors, working synergistically, produce high-risk situations (e.g., violence). For example, the presence of an inebriated family
member with a history of becoming violent when drinking, coupled with
a volatile adolescent, may lead to domestic violence. *Unpredictable crises* are unanticipated by the therapist or treatment team. Each type of
crisis has its own set of unique circumstances that place demands on, or
influence, the responsibilities of crisis team members. As crisis team
members gain clinical experience, the ratio of predictable to unpredictable crises should increase.

## Predictable Crises

After determining that a crisis is likely, the treatment team develops a
crisis plan and list of resources needed to implement the plan (see Figure
5.1). As families facing adversity ideally obtain emergency resources
from close interpersonal relationships and community ties, MST crisis
plans strive to tap indigenous sources of social support.

### DETERMINING RESOURCE NEEDS

Determining the resources needed to deal effectively with a predictable
crisis is predicated on a thorough understanding of the range of the
youth's previous responses to therapeutic interventions (e.g., therapeutic
holds, medications) and his or her physical size and strength. For example, a large imposing youth with a history of threatening his mother with
violence when she tries to provide appropriate discipline may have posed
little risk of physical harm to the mother in the past because she always
backed down in the face of her son's intimidation. If, however, the treatment team decides to place threatening behavior under extinction, the
youth may now become physically aggressive because the mother will no
longer be backing down. This youth's size also poses a number of other
concerns, the foremost of which is that larger youth have the potential of
inflicting more serious bodily injury than smaller youth. For pragmatic
reasons, larger and stronger youth often require more "manpower" to
intervene. Finally, knowing a youth's history of escalations and de-
escalations is also helpful in determining resource needs. For example,
youth with rapid escalations and de-escalations require fewer resources
than youth with prolonged escalations and de-escalations. These examples are just a few of the factors MST treatment teams must weigh in
determining resource needs. Factors associated with different types of
psychiatric emergencies and the strengths and needs of each system are
explored subsequently.

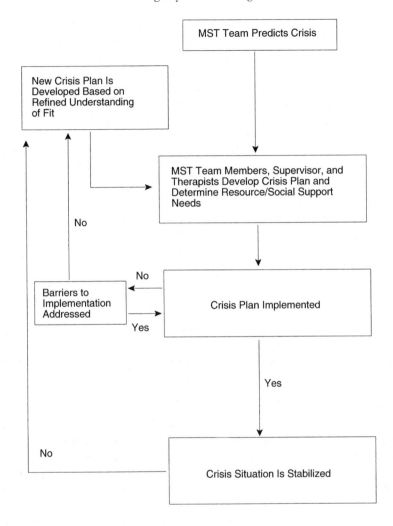

**FIGURE 5.1.** Predictable crisis.

## SOCIAL SUPPORTS

Social support resources fall along a continuum ranging from informal to formal and often play a key role in helping families overcome a crisis. Informal social supports are available in the immediate ecology (i.e., they are indigenous) and are part of the youth's or family's social network (e.g., family, friends, neighbors, coworkers). Moving along this continuum, the next level of resources would include those provided by community-based organizations such as schools, camps, churches, and neighborhood groups. The most formal social support resources are those provided by public agencies (e.g., social service, juvenile justice, mental health). To maintain ecological validity (Principle 8), crisis plans are designed to utilize supports on the informal portion of the continuum whenever possible. In general, the formal social supports are accessed only after all less formal options have been exhausted. Thus, if a child requires constant supervision (e.g., 24-hour supervision for the next 48–72 hours), the crisis team first uses available familial or indigenous supports before moving to treatment team or agency-based options. For example, the father may be responsible for monitoring the child at home between the hours of 2:00 P.M. and 9:00 P.M. and then is relieved by the MST crisis caseworker. The crisis caseworker may then monitor the child until 2:00 A.M. when the older sister gets home from work, who will then monitor the child until 6:00 A.M.

Unfortunately, the needs of some youth in crisis may exceed the capacity of indigenous, community, and MST crisis team resources. For example, an acutely suicidal child needing one-to-one supervision may exhaust the resources of a family, community, and crisis team over 4 or 5 days. After expending available supports, the treatment team may need to explore more formal resource options. The MST administrator is usually involved when the crisis plan calls for resources beyond the capacity of the family's social support network and the crisis team.

When clinical needs require formal resources, preference should be given to agencies or organizations that will allow MST treatment plans to follow the child. That is, the MST treatment team and family should remain directly involved in treatment such that therapeutic targets are consistent with MST's overarching treatment goals, MST treatment recommendations are valued and followed, and MST treatment teams and caregivers are consulted regarding the youth's care. Facilitating this level of involvement with formal resources requires (1) a collaborative relationship between the team and the agency providing formal resources and (2) a well-specified treatment plan. The MST administrator and supervisor must give final approval of all crisis plans involving formal resources.

## ASSIGNING TASKS TO CARRY OUT CRISIS PLANS

After a plan for dealing with the predictable crisis is developed and the resources and social supports needed to implement the plan are understood, the MST supervisor assigns specific individuals (e.g., crisis team members, caregivers) tasks and responsibilities for carrying out the treatment strategy (see Figure 5.1).

## Unpredictable Crises

Unpredictable crises (see Figure 5.2) often come to the attention of the therapist or crisis caseworker through a person in the community (e.g., caregivers, family members, teachers, social service personnel) reporting that the youth is imminently at risk of harm to self or others. At this point, the therapist or crisis caseworker arranges to meet directly with the youth and the informant. Upon arriving at the crisis scene, the team

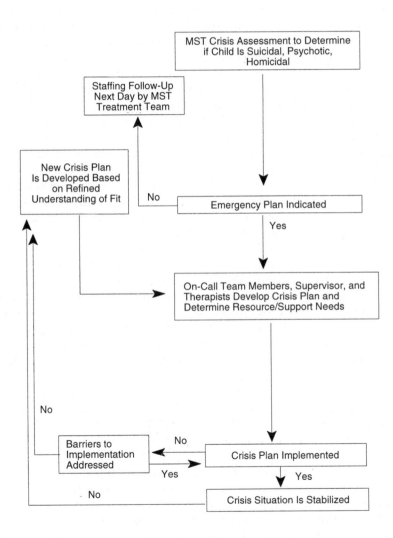

**FIGURE 5.2.** Unpredictable crisis.

member completes a MST crisis assessment (detailed subsequently) to determine if the youth is acutely at risk. If the youth is not at risk, a follow-up staff meeting is scheduled the next day with the treatment team to review the case. If the youth is acutely at risk of harm to self or others, steps are *immediately* taken to stabilize the crisis situation. For example, an MST therapist or crisis caseworker may be called to a school because of the suicidal threats of a client. The team member must quickly assess the environment (as specified subsequently), secure the child against harm to self or others (e.g., direct a teacher's aide to monitor the youth in a safe area, remove dangerous objects from the immediate environment), and then call the MST supervisor to develop a crisis plan. Immediately following crisis stabilization, the team member should consult with the MST supervisor and administrator to develop a continuing crisis plan. From this point on, the team follows the same algorithm developed for youth experiencing predictable crises. Thus, after a plan is developed and the resources and social supports needed to implement the plan are understood, the MST supervisor assigns specific individuals (e.g., treatment team members, caregivers) tasks and responsibilities to carry out the treatment strategy (see Figure 5.2).

In the remainder of this chapter, the critical elements of crisis assessment and intervention are highlighted. Consistent with the treatment philosophy of MST, interventions should address the known determinants of clinical problems across the ecologies of youths and families. The next section focuses on the correlates of serious emotional disturbance. Particular attention is paid to the correlates and risk factors associated with attempted and completed adolescent suicide, as this information largely drives the safety policy. The intent is not to provide a comprehensive review of childhood psychopathology, but to give the reader information gleaned from the relevant literature and clinical experience in addressing the mental health emergencies of youth with serious emotional disturbance in a community-based setting (Henggeler, Rowland, et al., 1997).

## CORRELATES OF SERIOUS EMOTIONAL DISTURBANCE: THE PLAYING FIELD OF MST CRISIS ASSESSMENT

A major concern that MST crisis teams must address in treating youth with serious emotional disturbance in a family and community-based setting is client safety. Client safety can only occur when treatment team members are aware of the factors that contribute to and exacerbate psychiatric emergencies. A growing body of empirical evidence has shown that serious antisocial behavior, childhood depression, adolescent suicide, and psychoses are associated with important characteristics of the individual youth and his or her family, peer relations, and community.

## Antisocial Behavior

Causal modeling studies have consistently found that antisocial behavior and serious behavioral problems are associated with factors related to individual, family, peer, school, and neighborhood characteristics. In a longitudinal evaluation of a national sample of adolescents, for example, Elliott, Huizinga, and Ageton (1985) found that association with deviant peers predicted serious criminal behavior 1 year later, and that family and school difficulties predicted association with deviant peers. Regarding violent delinquents, Fagan and Wexler (1987) found that the strongest predictors of violent offending were association with deviant peers and low school integration.

## Childhood Depression

Similarly, childhood depression has been associated with important characteristics of the youth and the multiple systems in which the youth is embedded. Individual characteristics associated with childhood depression include both biological and cognitive variables (Kazdin, 1983, 1990). For example, studies link childhood depression to a negative attributional style and hopelessness about the future (Gotlib, Lewinsohn, Seeley, Rohde, & Redner, 1993; Hops, Lewinsohn, Andrews, & Roberts, 1990; Quiggle, Garber, Panak, & Dodge, 1992). Family factors associated with childhood depression include parental resentment and rejection, lack of affection, disengagement, and discord (Crook, Raskin, & Eliot, 1981; Kashani, Burbach, & Rosenberg, 1988; Kaslow, Deering, & Racusin, 1994; Lefkowitz & Tesiny, 1984). Low trust, poor communication, alienation (Armsden & Greenberg, 1987; Armsden, McCauley, Greenberg, Burke, & Mitchell, 1990), and low social support (Barrera & Garrison-Jones, 1992) often mark the peer relations of depressed youngsters.

## Adolescent Psychosis

Most current etiological theories of childhood psychopathology (e.g., mood, thought, anxiety, personality, and substance abuse disorders) suggest individual characteristics (e.g., genetic loading, central nervous system dysfunctions, poor intellectual and social competence) interact with environmental stressors (e.g., pregnancy and birth complications, death of a parent, deviant family communication) to produce prodromal symptomatology (Mash & Dozois, 1996). For example, while genetic

and individual factors clearly play a role in the development of schizophrenia (Ninan & Mance, 1990), environmental factors such as family
communication style and exposure to stressors impact both the precipitation of the symptoms (Asarnow & Asarnow, 1996; Graham & Rutter,
1985) and the client's response to treatment (Leff, Kuipers, Berkowitz,
& Sturgeon, 1985; Vaughn & Leff, 1976).

## Adolescent Suicide

Suicidal behavior in adolescents also seems to be multidetermined. In a
study comparing adolescent suicide victims with suicidal inpatients,
Brent et al. (1988) found four risk factors were more prevalent among
adolescents with completed suicides: (1) diagnosis of bipolar disorder,
(2) affective disorder with comorbidity, (3) lack of previous mental
health treatment, and (4) availability of firearms. Firearms were more
likely to have been present in the homes of completers than attempters
and were the manner of death in the majority (70%) of suicide victims
whose homes contained firearms. Intoxication with alcohol also increases the danger of suicide attempt or completion. Data suggest that
these two risk factors (firearm availability and intoxication with alcohol)
may work synergistically to further increase the risk of suicide (Brent,
Perper, & Allman, 1987). These findings and the results of several other
studies support the removal of firearms from the home and limiting access to intoxicants as methods for diminishing risk of completed suicides
for youth (Boyd & Moscicki, 1986; Kellermann & Reay, 1986; Lester &
Murrell, 1980; Maris, 1991).

In addition, available data support the hypothesis that adolescent
suicide attempts are linked to aspects of the youth's larger ecology and
context as well as to individual symptomatology (Brent, Kolko, Allan, &
Brown, 1990; Brent et al., 1993; Cohen-Sandler, Berman, & King, 1982;
Gispert, Davis, Marsh, & Wheeler, 1987; Hawton, Osborn, O'Grady, &
Cole, 1982; Kotila & Lonnquist, 1989; Pfeffer et al., 1991). *Family variables* associated with suicide attempts include parent–child discord,
financial problems, loss of a parent or relative, poor family adaptive
functioning, and separation of the child from the home. *School and peer
variables* include poor functioning at school and alienation from peers.
*Associated individual symptoms* include affective disorder, suicidal ideation, low assertion, cognitive distortions, hostility, criminality, behavioral disorders, and substance abuse.

In summary, results from the child psychopathology literature
suggest that the types of problems exhibited by youths with serious emotional disturbance are multidetermined. Consequently, effective treatments and crisis responses (i.e., crisis plans) to the psychiatric emergen-

cies of youth with serious emotional disturbance should consider characteristics of the youth and the multiple systems in which he or she is embedded (e.g., family, peers, school, community).

## MST CRISIS ASSESSMENT

Consistent with MST treatment principles, the primary purpose of crisis assessment is to understand the fit of current behavior in light of its broader systemic context (e.g., family, peers, school, community). Crisis assessment, therefore, is a multidimensional process that identifies the unique strengths and needs of the youth and family and the fit of these strengths and needs with the resources of the family, indigenous supports, MST treatment team, and community. Thus, five broad domains of functioning, each with multiple levels, and the nature of the relations between these domains are investigated to determine factors that decrease (strengths) or increase (risk factors) the youth's risk of harm to self or others. These domains include the (1) individual youth, (2) family and immediate social ecology, (3) home/living environment, (4) peers, and (5) neighborhood and community.

### Individual Youth

At the level of individual functioning, the youth is assessed to determine his or her psychological state, medical status, and degree of cooperation. This information, in conjunction with the history of previous problematic behaviors, plays a crucial role in crisis planning. The psychological states most often encountered by team members during psychiatric emergencies fall into one of three categories: homicidal, suicidal, or psychotic. Several factors are associated with each of these states that may increase the risk of harm to self or others.

HOMICIDAL

Although much has been written about antisocial behavior and violence, few studies have actually examined factors associated with acute dangerousness (i.e., violence). Two types of studies have been used in predicting future violence: clinical and actuarial. Investigations examining clinical predictions of dangerousness have found that "at best," the accuracy of this method falls below 50% (Melton, Petrila, Poythress, & Slobogin, 1997). Actuarial and statistical methods of predicting dangerousness have fared somewhat better than clinical predictions, but their accuracy is also unsatisfactory (Gottfredson & Gottfredson, 1988; Quinsey &

Maguire, 1986). A consistent finding among both types of predictions is the high false positive rate (i.e., predicting someone will be violent who in fact does not become violent) these methods produce. For example, across clinical and actuarial studies the false positive rate has ranged from 19% to 99% (Melton et al., 1997).

Despite the apparent shortcomings of clinical and actuarial methods of predicting dangerousness, MST treatment teams must still decide whether youth with serious emotional disturbance experiencing a psychiatric emergency should be stabilized in a community-based or more restrictive setting. Two options available for assessing a client's dangerousness, based on the extant literature, include examination of (1) risk factors associated with a particular individual who belongs to a class of individuals whose violence potential is known (i.e., the actuarial approach), and (2) examination of personal and situational factors (i.e., the contextual factors approach) contributing to the client's previous violent behavior or episodes (Melton et al., 1997).

*Actuarial Approach.* Several demographic characteristics are associated with future violence, including (adapted from Monahan, 1981a, 1981b):

1. *Prior arrest for a violent crime:* The probability of future violence increases with each subsequent arrest.
2. *Age:* A strong correlation exists between age and criminal activity such that violence peaks in the late teens and early 20s. Youths with a young age of first arrest and chronic juvenile offenders are at greater risk for committing a violent act.
3. *Sex:* In general, males are much more violent than females.
4. *Race:* African Americans and other nonwhites commit disproportionately more crimes than Caucasians.
5. *Socioeconomic status (SES) and employment:* Low SES, employment instability, and less educational attainment (poor educational achievement among youth) are associated with violent offending.
6. *Opiate and alcohol abuse:* Substance abuse is associated with violence.
7. *Low IQ:* The lower the IQ, the more likely a person is to engage in violent behavior.
8. *Residential stability:* Violence is more likely among those who move frequently.
9. *Family environment:* High family conflict and low family warmth are associated with serious offending.
10. *Peer associations:* Association with deviant peers is one of the strongest predictors of juvenile offending.

This list of demographic characteristics is of minimal utility for an MST treatment team whose clientele consists primarily of poor and disenfranchised minorities living in lower SES urban communities. Of more utility for predicting future violence is an examination of the contextual factors associated with the individual client's previous violent behavior.

*Contextual Approach.* Situational factors associated with violent behavior include:

1. *Recency, frequency, and severity of previous violent acts:* An individual whose pattern of violent behavior is escalating in terms of severity and frequency is at higher risk of subsequent violence than if his or her violent behavior is declining.
2. *Environmental stressors:* Situational factors such as family stress or loss can contribute to higher risk. For example, a person is more likely to become violent when a close interpersonal relationship ends.
3. *Availability of victims:* Individuals are much more dangerous when their previous violence has been directed toward a broad range of victims, or when they have committed multiple assaults on a narrow range of victims who are currently available in their environment.
4. *Availability of weapons:* Availability of weapons significantly increases the risk of violence.

Thus, as with all MST assessments, the crisis team must determine the fit of the youth's behavior. In particular, team members must pay attention to the contextual factors in the current environment that may either increase or decrease that youth's risk for violence.

## SUICIDAL

When a client communicates an intent to commit suicide or is considering suicide, the members of the treatment team should immediately assess factors that place the client at imminent risk of harm to self. Working with adult populations, Linehan (1993) categorized factors associated with imminent risk of suicide into direct indices and indirect indices.

*Direct Indices.* Direct indices of imminent risk for suicide include:

1. *Suicidal ideation:* The team member should assess the frequency, intensity, and duration of suicidal thoughts. As the frequency, intensity, and/or duration of suicidal thoughts increases, the risk of harm also in-

creases. For example, a person who constantly thinks about suicide is at higher risk than a person who thinks about suicide less frequently. Likewise, a person who devotes considerable cognitive energy (intensity) to controlling suicidal thoughts is at higher risk than a person who devotes minimal cognitive energy to this task.

2. *Lethality of suicide threat:* For a team member to estimate the risk of harm a suicidal patient poses, the therapist must know what suicidal methods are likely to produce a lethal outcome (Smith, Conroy, & Ehler, 1984). Common methods of suicide in order of lethality are "(1) firearms and explosives, (2) jumping from high places, (3) cutting and piercing vital organs, (4) hanging, (5) drowning (cannot swim), (6) poisoning (solids and liquids), (7) cutting and piercing nonvital organs, (8) drowning (can swim), (9) poisoning (gases), and (10) analgesic and soporific substances" (cited in Linehan, 1993, p. 481). For adolescents, the modal method for completed suicide is firearms and explosives (Berman & Jobes, 1992).

3. *Suicide planning and/or preparation:* Suicidal ideas, talk, and preparation are evident in most suicides. For example, in approximately 80% of suicides, presuicidal clues included having a specific plan (i.e., when, how), giving away valued possessions, discussing death or suicide, changing normal routines (e.g., missing work, school, or church uncharacteristically), drinking heavily, abusing drugs, and acting out sexually (Maris, 1991). Thus, crisis team members must question clients about suicidal plans and methods (availability, accessibility, lethality), if they left a suicide note, and whether they have taken any precautions against discovery or intervention (Linehan, 1993). Of course, clients who are unwilling to provide this information are at increased risk to harm themselves.

4. *Previous suicide attempt:* The rate of suicide in the general population is approximately 1 per 10,000 (or 0.01%), while the rate for previous suicide attempters is 1 in 10 (or 10%). Thus, a history of suicide attempts greatly increases the risk of suicide (Maris, 1991).

*Indirect Indices.* Indirect indices of imminent risk for suicide include:

1. *Client in high-risk population:* Older white males (and among adolescents, older adolescents) and people with mental disorders, with affective illness, or with a family history of suicide fall into high-risk populations.

2. *Recent change or loss of social support:* People who have experienced loss of social support (e.g., death of a loved one), stressful life events (e.g., failure at school or work, financial problems, re-

lationship discord, conflict, a threat of imprisonment), or discharge from a psychiatric hospital are at increased risk of completing a suicide attempt.

3. *Dissatisfaction with treatment.*
4. *Hopelessness, anger, or both.*
5. *Recent medical treatment or physical illness.*
6. *Indirect references to own death, making arrangements for death.*
7. *Abrupt clinical change, either positive or negative.*

To summarize, therapists must examine individual symptoms of the youth as well as contextual factors in determining risk for suicide. Individual symptoms that suggest youth are at higher risk include affective illness (particularly bipolar affective disorder), substance use, hopelessness, frequent or intense suicidal ideations, past suicide attempts, and preparation for death. As discussed subsequently, environmental factors that place youth at risk include access to a weapon, family discord and conflict, loss, poor academic functioning, and alienation from peers. An accurate assessment of risk for suicide can only be performed when clinicians understand the fit of the client's current suicidal ideation and individual and contextual factors that promote or attenuate symptoms.

## PSYCHOTIC

When working with a youth or family member exhibiting symptoms of psychosis, the impact of these symptoms on treatment plan conceptualization and implementation must be recognized. As with any other type of crisis situation, the treatment team must attempt to gain an understanding of the fit of the psychotic symptoms within the individual's context. Thus, team members will need to understand the psychological, biological, and social/environmental settings in which the symptoms developed. As the word *psychosis* can be interpreted differently by individual clinicians depending on their training and clinical experiences, this section begins by defining this term to ensure consensus.

The term *psychosis* means loss of contact with reality (Torrey, 1988) and implies a serious disturbance in an individual's reality testing as reflected by specific pathological signs (Volkmar, 1996). These signs often come in the form of *hallucinations, delusions,* or *thought disturbances. Hallucinations* are sensory perceptions that are not based in reality. These may occur in any sensory modality (sight, taste, touch, sound, or smell). Examples of hallucinations include seeing snakes or hearing voices. *Delusions* are fixed false beliefs that are held despite contradictory evidence. For instance, someone may believe he or she is receiving special messages from the radio or being followed by the FBI. *Thought disorders* are best detected by listening to a person's speech, both its pattern and content. Often, individuals with a thought disorder will demonstrate speech that is not well formed, logical, or coherent— rapidly jumping from one idea to the next, needlessly repeating the same thought, or including too many details and irrelevant pieces of information. In extreme cases, the speech of psychotic individuals may be incoherent or impossible to follow (American Psychiatric Association, 1994).

Clinically, the term *psychosis* suggests schizophrenia, yet symptoms of psychosis may reflect several different medical or psychiatric conditions. From a psychiatric perspective, psychotic symptoms may present as part of a mood disorder (depression, mania), obsessive–compulsive disorder, dissociative state, posttraumatic stress disorder, personality disorder (schizoid, schizotypal, paranoid, or borderline), schizoaffective disorder (concurrent symptoms of schizophrenia and depression or mania), or pervasive developmental disorder (autism, Rett's disorder, Asperger's syndrome, or childhood disintegrative disorders) depending on the age of onset and associated symptoms (McClellan & Werry, 1994; Tolbert, 1996).

*Medical Conditions.* Several medical conditions may be accompanied by psychotic symptoms. In particular, the clinical syndromes of *delirium* and *dementia* may present with features similar to psychosis. Differentiating these syndromes from psychosis significantly impacts the formulation of treatment plans. *Delirium* is a rapidly developing disorder of disturbed attention or consciousness that changes with time. Characteristics that help differentiate delirium from psychosis include fluctuating level of consciousness, sudden change in attention span, increased distractibility, disorientation, memory impairment, and incoherence. Delirium is almost always caused by a medical problem (e.g., infection, low blood sugar, drug reaction, trauma); hence, immediate medical attention is indicated (Tomb, 1995). *Dementia* usually develops slowly and results from a broad loss of intellectual functions due to diffuse organic disease of the brain. Over time, someone with dementia may develop symptoms of memory loss, intellectual impairment, language impairment, compromised judgment, and changes in mood and personality (American Psychiatric Association, 1994). Thus, for individuals with psychotic symptoms, clinicians must determine whether the psychosis is occurring within the context of one of these conditions to ensure that appropriate care is provided.

Other medical conditions that may be accompanied by psychotic symptoms include substance intoxication or withdrawal. Intoxication with sedative hypnotics (e.g., alcohol, benzodiazepines, barbiturates), hallucinogens (e.g., LSD, PCP, cannabis), stimulants (e.g., amphetamines, cocaine), or inhalants and anabolic steroids may precipitate psychotic symptoms. Withdrawal from stimulants (e.g., cocaine) and sedative hypnotics such as alcohol, barbiturates, and benzodiazepines (e.g., Valium, Librium, Ativan, Serax) may precipitate psychotic symptoms; importantly, withdrawal from sedative hypnotics may be life-threatening. Thus, if an individual has known or suspected dependence on sedative hypnotics and presents with visual hallucinations, tactile hallucinations, tremulousness, nausea, vomiting, or signs of delirium, immediate medical attention is indicated (Tomb, 1995). *Seizure disorders* (temporal lobe focus), *brain tumors, heavy metal toxins,* and *degenerative neurological disorders* may also precipitate psychotic symptoms (McClellan & Werry, 1994).

*Environmental Factors.* While genetic and biological factors almost always play a role in the development of psychotic symptoms, environmental factors often contribute to the precipitation of symptoms, relapse rates, and level of functioning between episodes of illness (Ninan & Mance, 1990). For example, family factors such as expressed emotion (e.g., criticism, hostility, overinvolvement) are associated with higher relapse rates in schizophrenia (Leff &Vaughn, 1981). Environmental stressors may also contribute to the precipitation of symptoms, whereas adequate social resources have been associated with good prognosis in individuals with either affective or schizophrenic forms of psychosis (Erickson, Beiser, Iacono, Fleming, & Lin, 1989).

*Medication.* Even if psychotic symptoms are considered to be psychiatric in nature, a physician will need to be involved in the care of this individual to rule out medical etiology and to consider psychotropic medications. Currently, neuroleptics have documented efficacy in the treatment of adults with psychosis (Davis, Comaty, & Janicak, 1987). While fewer studies support the use of neuroleptics in children and adolescents, several investigations have shown that adolescents respond similarly to adults (Campbell, Gonzalez, Ernst, Silva, & Werry, 1993; Spencer, Kafantaris, Padron-Gayol, Rosenberg, & Campbell, 1992). Thus, medication will most likely be part of a comprehensive treatment plan for individuals with psychosis.

In summary, when presented with a youth or adult in the community who is exhibiting psychotic symptoms, crisis team members will need to develop an understanding of the psychological, medical, and environmental underpinnings of the presenting problem. If symptoms of delirium, dementia, substance intoxication, withdrawal, or other medical conditions are present, immediate medical attention should be sought. New onset psychosis in individuals that pose a significant risk of harm to self or others will probably need closer monitoring and evaluation than is provided in most community settings. A plan to stabilize an individual in the community is more likely to be appropriate if there is a known history of psychosis, adequate supports, and the treatment team understands the fit of the psychotic behavior and can impact the precipitants. For example, a youth with a past history of schizophrenia who presents with a thought disorder and paranoid delusions after 2 weeks of medication noncompliance may be able to be treated in the community if the fit of the medication noncompliance is addressed and appropriate monitoring and supervision can be provided.

For all youth presenting in crisis, the team members must consider the youth's current medical status and the role physical illness may play in the presenting problem. The team child psychiatrist should be consulted whenever youth present with unusual physical symptoms or behaviors, or when they have a current or past history of significant medical problems (e.g., diabetes, head trauma). Finally, the youth's degree of cooperation and history of previous behaviors should be integrated into the team's assessment.

## Family and Immediate Social Environment

Crisis team members need to develop an understanding of who is in the youth's family and social ecology, their role in the current crisis, and their availability to assist in stabilizing the situation. When these factors are determined, those individuals selected to be crisis stabilizers must be evaluated to ensure that they are able to perform this task.

### COMPOSITION OF THE IMMEDIATE SOCIAL ENVIRONMENT

The MST team starts the assessment of the immediate social environment by identifying all significant biological and nonbiological caregivers, siblings, and extended family members (e.g., aunts, uncles, grandparents, etc.). Next, individuals outside the family who have significant impact on youth and family functioning are identified. These individuals might include friends (of both youth and caregiver), teachers, pastors, neighbors, and coworkers of caregivers.

*Individuals Directly Involved in the Crisis.* After determining who comprises the youth's immediate social ecology, team members assess the relationship of those persons available to the child (e.g., parent, guardian, sibling, aunt, cousin), their role in the current crisis (e.g., stabilizing influence vs. an instigator), and their physical proximity to the child (i.e., access to the child). By this time, team clinicians must be attempting to understand the fit of the behavior precipitating the crisis and the roles individuals involved in the crisis played. Thus, the psychological state of these individuals (e.g., depressed, psychotic, intoxicated, stable) as well as a gross sense of their intellectual functioning will need to be determined before crisis stabilization plans can be developed.

*Determining Who Is Available in the Immediate Social Environment to Help Stabilize the Crisis.* When crisis team members understand who is in the youth's natural ecology and the role they play (if any) in the current crisis, team members can work with the youth and family to identify who on their list can provide the resources needed to stabilize the crisis. Thus, for a youth who needs more monitoring, an important task will be to find adults who are capable of supervising the youth.

When someone is going to monitor or care for a youth, the MST team must take several steps to ensure that the selected caregiver is appropriate for the assignment. Individuals who help stabilize the crisis must have several characteristics, including:

1. *Understands the gravity of the situation* as demonstrated by words or action. For example, the stabilizer can articulate the potential outcomes associated with the current situation.
2. *Cares* about what happens to the client.
3. *Is emotionally stable*—for example, the stabilizer is able to remain calm while others in the environment are not.
4. *Is willing to participate* in the crisis plan for a specified period of time (e.g., for the next 24 to 48 hours).
5. *Agrees that the crisis plan is viable.*
6. *Possesses cognitive and/or physical abilities* equal to or greater than those needed to complete the task.

This list has been incorporated into the MST Crisis Team Safety Checklist (Rowland, Cunningham, & Kruesi, 2001) (Figure 5.3) to assist clinicians in remembering these points during the assessment. Once they understand a youth's family and immediate social ecology, MST clinicians need to assess the youth's home or living environment.

## Home/Living Environment

Assessment of the home/living environment as a possible treatment site considers several factors, including the presence of weapons and other

**FIGURE 5.3.** Intake Crisis Safety Checklist.

*First Assessment of Site*

This version of the checklist is to be done with each new site the youth lives in and is to be followed up with a Second Assessment within 1 week, earlier if indicated.

Client name: _____ Site of assessment: _____ Date: _____

GUNS

***Ensure the youth and siblings are not present when interviewing family concerning guns.***

Ask all caregivers if guns are present in the home. Were guns present? Y____ / N____

***If guns are present immediately call the supervisor. Do not leave the home until you have called the supervisor and established a safety plan.***

If guns were present, was the supervisor called? Y____ / N____
If guns were present, what plan was followed?
Family removed gun _____
    If gun was removed, where was it placed? _____
Family placed lock on gun _____ (gun must be unloaded for this to be safe)
Family put gun in locker or lock box _____
    If placed in locker or lock box, where are all keys to lock? _____

Please note below all actions taken to ensure youth does not have access to weapon. If the weapon goes to the house of a family member, actions should be taken to secure it from use by this youth or other children in that home.

_____
_____
_____
_____

Does youth have access to guns in the community (e.g., friend or family member with gun)? Y____ / N____
Please note below all actions taken to limit youth's access to these weapons (e.g., having relatives dispose of weapons, limiting access to peer with gun). _____
_____
_____

OTHER DANGEROUS WEAPONS OR OBJECTS

Speak with the therapist or supervisor and find out the following:
Does the youth have past history of (check all that apply)
    ❑ Suicide attempts
    ❑ Homicide attempts
    ❑ Assault or aggression toward others

List all weapons or items used in these attempts in the space below. Follow by checking if these items were found in the home, and indicate plan for removal or ensuring safety. Use medication section below to document disposal or storage of medication.

    ❑ _____ (found Y / N) Disposal _____
    ❑ _____ (found Y / N) Disposal _____
    ❑ _____ (found Y / N) Disposal _____
    ❑ _____ (found Y / N) Disposal _____

## MEDICATIONS

Ask caregiver what medications the youth takes. List the names of the medications and the quantity in the house below.

Ask caregiver if you may go through the medicine cabinet. This is so that you can help the parent ensure the youth's future safety. If youth has a history of suicide attempt by medication ingestion or significant impulsivity, stress the importance of this search. You should also ask to see medication bottles, as this will help you see name and amount in bottle.

When filling out actions taken, if possible describe using one of the following terms.

1. Medication disposed (e.g., flushed down toilet).
2. Medication removed from home with caregiver's consent (list where placed by whom).
3. Medication supply placed in locked box.
4. Medication supply placed in safe place without youth access (describe).
5. N/A—no action taken, await supervisor's input.
6. Attempted to take action, parent refused, supervisor/therapist notified.

| *Medication* | *Quantity* | *Action taken* |
|---|---|---|
| _____ | _____ | _____ |
| _____ | _____ | _____ |
| _____ | _____ | _____ |
| _____ | _____ | _____ |

Ask caregiver what medications the caregiver and any other family members take. List the names of the medications and the quantity in the house below. Be careful to ask about antidepressants, sleeping pills, and heart medications.

| *Medication* | *Quantity* | *Action taken* |
|---|---|---|
| _____ | _____ | _____ |
| _____ | _____ | _____ |
| _____ | _____ | _____ |
| _____ | _____ | _____ |

Ask to see any general medications used to relieve pain. List the names of the medications and the quantity available in the house in the space below. Here, you are looking to see if the family has large quantities of aspirin or Tylenol (acetaminophen), which can be potentially lethal.

| *Medication* | *Quantity* | *Action taken* |
|---|---|---|
| _____ | _____ | _____ |
| _____ | _____ | _____ |
| _____ | _____ | _____ |
| _____ | _____ | _____ |

If the youth has a history of suicide attempt by medication ingestion, call the supervisor and report the quality and quantity of medications you have found. Record what actions you take concerning each medication.

| _____ | _____ | _____ |
|---|---|---|
| _____ | _____ | _____ |

(*continued* )

**FIGURE 5.3.** (*continued*)

<u>DRUG USE/ALCOHOL</u>

Ask all caregivers about alcohol use in the home (youth and other family members). Ask caregiver to tell you what alcohol is in the home (including beer and wine) and where it is stored. List name and place stored below.

_____    _____    _____

_____    _____    _____

Ask caregiver about youth substance use and describe the drug and how often youth uses it below:

_____    _____    _____

_____    _____    _____

If youth has history by parent or youth report of using drugs, search the youth's room (with parent's permission) for drugs.

History? Y_____ / N _____ Permission to search given? Y _____ / N _____

Results of search: list name of drug, amount, and what was done to dispose of the drug. Caregivers should dispose of the drug in your presence (e.g., by flushing it down the toilet). Actions taken should be described using the following categories:

1. Drug removed (describe name of person who removed it and how it was disposed of)
2. Drug not removed, supervisor called

***Never take illegal substances or drug paraphernalia into your own possession.***

***Drug***                          ***Quantity***                      ***Action taken***

_____    _____    _____

_____    _____    _____

<u>ENVIRONMENT</u>

Please use the space below to describe anything in the environment that is a concern given what you know about the youth's history. This may include things like a broken window in the living room, a brother's weight set, or a toolbox nearby. Also include things in the near vicinity of the house such as a crack house next-door.

_____

_____

_____

_____

_____

<u>BEFORE LEAVING</u>

If there is anything that you have found in the safety check that you feel may pose significant risk for the youth or other family members, call the supervisor now concerning this if you have not already done so. If the supervisor does not return your call, contact the MST psychiatrist on call and develop a plan before leaving the home.

Note this concern and any actions taken that you have not already noted above.

_____

_____

_____

_____

_____

_____

Bring this checklist to the next supervision with a photocopy for your file.
Done? Y_____ N_____

Discuss findings with therapist and supervisor in supervision.
Done? Y _____ N _____

**File original copy in chart ASAP!!!!**

**Go to home and complete follow-up assessment (INTAKE CRISIS SAFETY CHECKLIST *Second Assessment*) within 1 week of this assessment—sooner if indicated during supervision. *The Second Assessment* must always be done regardless of findings unless youth moves to another site before it is completed. If this occurs, complete another *First Assessment* of this new site.**

suicidal or homicidal means and the availability of a contained place where the youth can be monitored. In light of the complexity inherent in crisis assessment of the home/living environment as a possible treatment site, a Crisis Team Safety Checklist (Figure 5.3) has been developed to help MST clinicians decide upon the best treatment site, and follow-up checklists are used to provide continuing safety monitoring (Rowland et al., 2001).

WEAPONS

The MST team must complete a thorough assessment of the living environment for the presence of weapons and other potentially lethal methods for causing harm to self or others. This task is often performed by the crisis caseworker but may be performed by any team member when indicated. Thus, for example, if the treatment team decides and the caretaker agrees that the youth should stay with a neighbor for a few days following serious familial conflicts, the neighbor's home becomes the crisis treatment site, and the crisis caseworker searches the neighbor's home for weapons. Absence of a weapon means weapons *were not found* in the client's immediate living environment. That is, a team member and caregiver *have searched* the entire living environment and failed to find weapons. Although the presence of an unloaded and secured (i.e., locked away) firearm may seem to pose little risk, such "secured" weapons have been used in subsequent suicides and homicides (Brent et al., 1987, 1988). Thus, the presence of firearms, even if unloaded and secured, makes that living environment unsuitable as a treatment site option.

## PRESENCE OF OTHER SUICIDAL OR HOMICIDAL MEANS

In addition to looking for firearms, team members must assess for the presence of other means of hurting oneself or others. Such means include prescription and nonprescription medications, automobile in an enclosed space, rope/sheets, sharp objects (e.g., knives, razor blades), and bathtubs. When potentially dangerous medications are present, a team member must gather information concerning the name of the medication, number of pills present, dosage, how secured, and who has access. This information, along with a plan for placing the medication in a safe place that is not accessible to the youth, is recorded on the Crisis Team Safety Checklist (Figure 5.3). In particular, team members are taught to pay careful attention to heart medications, sedatives, and antidepressants, as well as to some common drugs such as aspirin and acetaminophen (Tylenol). The child psychiatrist should be consulted if team members are unsure of the potential lethality of a medication. In general, the team must combine common sense and its knowledge of the youth and family's past history to determine if routine household objects such as bathtubs and sheets pose a significant risk for a particular youth. While guns and sharp knives must always be removed from the home, other routine household objects (medications, scissors) may be secured or left in place depending upon the youth's presentation, past history, and environmental factors. Of course, team members should always be cautious and err on the side of safety if uncertain of the risks posed by various aspects of the environment.

## CONTAINED PLACE FOR YOUTH TO BE MONITORED

If a child requires close monitoring (e.g., one-to-one supervision), he or she should be monitored in a comfortable room on a lower floor with one door and secured windows. The monitoring room must be clear of dangerous, large, and sharp objects.

After the family and home environment have been assessed, the MST clinician must attempt to gain an understanding of any other aspects of the youth's ecology that may contribute to the current crisis situation.

## Peers

When assessing peer involvement, the MST team must consider the direct and indirect roles peers may play in the current crisis. Peers may directly impact the crisis in a negative way if they are a coaggressor with the adolescent (e.g., gang member) or a supplier of means (e.g., drugs, guns). Alternatively, peers may directly impact the crisis in a positive way by encouraging prosocial activities or providing emotional support. Examples of indirect involvement include those in which a peer has modeled the current behavior (e.g., suicide, violence) or serves as the source of an argument. Given the strong influence that peer relations play in adolescent development, the MST team should consider the role of peers in facilitating treatment. Thus, appropriate peers may be utilized (with youth and caregiver consent) to report imminent risk, identify high-risk situations, help prevent the youth's access to harm, or mobilize youth social support resources.

After the family, home environment, and peer group have been assessed, the MST clinician must gain an understanding of any other aspects of the youth's ecology that may contribute to the current crisis situation. In this final aspect of the assessment, the MST clinician should consider the neighborhood and community in which the crisis occurred.

### Neighborhood and Community

Here, the clinician examines the resources or barriers in the youth's community that could impact crisis treatment. Thus, if the house next door to the youth's home is a "crack house" frequented by drug dealers, this will influence the precautions taken by team members when they go to and from the home. Or if limiting the youth's access to weapons is difficult due to the sheer number of guns in the community, steps may need to be taken to monitor the youth more closely. On the other hand, churches, health clinics, schools, parks, and other community-based programs may provide valuable resources that can be used in the crisis treatment plan.

When complete, information obtained in the assessment will identify factors in the domains of the youth, family, home, peers, neighborhood, and community that decrease (strengths) or increase (barriers) the youth's risk of harm to self or others. The next section outlines how this information is synthesized to facilitate decisions regarding the initial placement of the child or adolescent.

## INTEGRATING RISK FACTORS
## TO DETERMINE PLACEMENT SITE

To create a treatment plan from the information obtained during the assessment, team members must understand not only the specific factors that decrease or increase the youth's risk of harm to self or others, but how these factors interact with each other to impact the youth's behavior. In other words, the fit of risk behavior within the youth's broader systemic context must be understood. Thus, for example, two youth with almost the same presentations of intense suicidal ideation may precipitate two very different treatment plans based on their respective contexts. To help clinicians develop an appropriate treatment plan, the MST team should denote the qualities of the five assessed domains (individual, family/social ecology, living environment, peers, neighborhood/community) as high risk or low risk. While somewhat categorical, completing such a checklist may provide a framework that team members can use when discussing and developing safety plans.

Based on the risk factors described previously, Table 5.1 presents the individual, family, and environmental factors that are indicative of high versus low risk. To create a treatment plan from the information obtained in the assessment, team members must understand not only the specific factors that decrease or increase the youth's risk of harm to self or others, but how these people and systems interface with each other to impact the youth's behavior. Crisis team members must weigh the combination of risk factors across categories present during a crisis when determining risk. In addition, team members must make decisions regarding where (treatment site) and how (crisis treatment modalities) to treat the youth, while identifying and procuring available community supports.

Clinicians should use the Form for MST Crisis Assessment of Youth, Family, and Environment (Figure 5.4) to help conceptualize the risks and strengths of the youth, family, home, peers, and community. The combination of risks and strengths across these systems is used to guide decisions concerning the appropriate treatment site and modality. Thus, by using the categorical system described in Table 5.1 for assigning low or high risk, team members can develop a better sense of where strengths and barriers exist. Using this system the team can conceptualize a variety of combinations ranging from a high-risk youth with least appropriate family response and most dangerous living environment to a low-risk youth with most appropriate family response and least dangerous living environment. As most youth will fall somewhere between the two extremes of this continuum, team decisions will have to be based on the relative strengths and weaknesses in each system.

### Individual Youth

A youth who is at high risk will need a family environment and treatment site that can accommodate his or her risk factors safely. Thus,

**TABLE 5.1. Individual, Family, and Environmental Factors Indicative of High Risk**

Highest-risk adolescent

1. Intense suicidal or homicidal ideation.
2. Current lethal plans with access to means.
3. History of previous attempts.
4. Isolation, precautions against discovery, suicide note.
5. Currently intoxicated, psychotic, manic, very anxious, or depressed.
6. Uncooperative with therapist, family, and crisis treatment plan.

Highest-risk family context

1. Caregivers or family members directly and negatively involved in the current crisis.
2. Caregiver emotionally unstable due to psychopathology (e.g., psychoses, substance abuse, depression, etc.).
3. Caregiver doesn't appear to understand the seriousness of the situation.
4. Caregiver doesn't appear to care about what happens to the child.
5. Caregiver unwilling to commit to time-defined involvement with the crisis plan.
6. Caregiver unconvinced that crisis treatment plan will work.
7. Caregiver unable to follow through with the crisis treatment plan because of limited cognitive abilities.

Most dangerous environment

1. Presence of weapons, specifically *guns*.
2. Second-story or higher monitoring room.
3. Unsecured monitoring room.
4. Unmonitored.
5. Ongoing verbal and/or physical conflict and aggression in the environment.
6. Ongoing substance abuse in the environment.

Lower-risk adolescent

1. A nonlethal plan with no access to means.
2. No previous history of suicide attempts.
3. No current intoxication, psychosis, mania, or severe psychopathology.
4. Some level of cooperation with therapist, family, and crisis treatment plan.

Lower-risk family context

1. Caregiver or family member involved in the crisis but able to detach enough to discuss the situation rationally.
2. Caregiver or family member emotionally stable.
3. Caregiver or family member understands the seriousness of the situation.
4. Caregiver or family member cares about what happens to the youth.
5. Caregiver or family member willing to commit to time-defined involvement with crisis treatment plan.
6. Family or family member has some faith that the crisis treatment plan can work and is committed to the plan.

Safer home/living environment (treatment site)

1. No guns.
2. No other weapons.
3. First-story monitoring room.

Crisis Assessment Form of Youth in Multisystemic Therapy

| System | Risk |
|---|---|

Highest                                              Lowest

Youth

Most Appropriate                              Least Appropriate

Family

Most Dangerous                       Least Dangerous Environment

(Home/peer/community)

**Crisis Treatment Site:**

**Crisis Treatment Modalities:**

**Crisis Treatment Community Supports:**

**FIGURE 5.4.** Form for MST Crisis Assessment of Youth, Family, and Environment.

when a youth is at high risk due to psychopathology such as depression, mania, psychosis, or intoxication, the team will need to decide if the strengths in the family and living environment can offset individual risk factors.

High-risk youth with high-risk family or environmental contexts are more likely to require an out-of-home placement. To increase ecological validity, the least restrictive community-based site (e.g., home of someone in the extended family, friends, respite foster care) is preferable to more restrictive placements (e.g., shelters, psychiatric hospitals, jails), yet safety must be the team's first concern. Thus, when faced with a youth with high-risk symptoms, the team must determine what family and environmental contexts are needed to keep this youth safe, and then look for the least restrictive setting that can provide these protective factors. Thus, a youth who presents with severe manic symptoms and agitation whose behavior is not responsive to the usual behavioral contingencies that can be administered in the community may require several days of psychiatric hospitalization for rapid stabilization with medications before returning to a community context. Yet another youth who presents with high-risk symptoms such as severe depression, suicidal ideation, and a suicide plan, and who lives in a high-risk family environment, may be able to be treated in the community (e.g., at grandmother's house) if appropriate supports and monitoring can be provided in an environment that is safe.

## Family and Social Environment

When the youth is living in a high-risk family context, the team should decide if acute interventions can be implemented to alter this context and diminish the risk. If not, the youth must be removed from this environment until interventions that target risk factors can be developed and implemented. For example, a youth who feels homicidal toward a stepfather may be able to be maintained safely in the home if the stepfather agrees to stay out of the home for a few days while the therapist works with family members to develop a better long-term solution.

Sometimes a safer family environment may be created by increasing supports from the natural ecology or crisis team. Thus, if a caregiver is unable to monitor a youth or follow through with a treatment plan, having someone from the natural ecology (e.g., grandfather, aunt) or treatment team stay in the home and provide monitoring and structure may diminish the risk of the family/social environment to the extent that the youth can remain in the home. If a safe family environment cannot be created for the youth, out-of-home placement will be required until the family risk factors are decreased or a substitute caregiver can be found. As always, the least restrictive community-based site that can safely accommodate the youth should be used.

## Home and Living Environment (Including Peers and Neighborhood)

When aspects of the home, peer group or neighborhood create a high risk situation for the youth, the team must decide if acute interventions can be conducted to diminish the risk. If not, the youth should be removed from this environment until interventions that target the risk can be developed and implemented. For example, if a youth is involved in criminal activity with delinquent peers that live nearby, he or she may be able to be maintained safely in the home if appropriate supervision is provided. On the other hand, an adolescent who lives in a home with ongoing physical aggression and conflict will need to be removed if this threatens his or her safety. As always, care should be taken to place the youth in the least restrictive community-based site that can safely accommodate his or her needs.

## CRISIS MANAGEMENT: TREATMENT INTERVENTIONS

An important goal of crisis management is to de-escalate any agitated or emotionally labile clients. Treatment options to de-escalate an agitated client include individual crisis therapy (e.g., empathy, unconditional positive regard), behavioral interventions, and pharmacotherapy. Criteria for selecting an option include (1) the history of successful interventions under similar conditions (e.g., if a behavioral intervention previously worked under similar conditions, that intervention is incorporated into the current crisis intervention plan), (2) the presence of organic symptomatology such as psychosis or mania, and (3) systemic strengths (resources) available to address the current crisis (e.g., the family's ability to intervene in de-escalating the crisis situation).

### Elements of Crisis Management Plans

Whatever crisis treatment modality is chosen, the team strategy must include preventive actions to safely manage client risk of harm to self or others, consultation with the MST supervisor, and adherence to the crisis treatment plan. Generally, preventive activities seek to (1) negate opportunities to harm self or others (e.g., removing the youth from a high-risk setting), (2) restrict access to homicidal or suicidal means (e.g., guns, medications), (3) intensify treatment (e.g., increasing amount of contact via more frequently scheduled appointments or phone contacts), (4) mobilize social supports and/or warn potential victims, and (5) increase supervision and monitoring (e.g., youth should not be left alone).

The treatment team must always consult the MST supervisor during a psychiatric emergency. Clinically, consultation allows the supervisor to ensure that the crisis treatment plan makes sense within the context of the overall MST treatment plan and that it ensures the safety of the client, family, and community. Also, as crisis situations are often volatile, communication allows the supervisor to act as a "second opinion" or sounding board for the therapist concerning the possible fit of the current crisis and interventions that may be indicated. Administratively, the supervisor must ensure that the therapist or crisis caseworker is handling the crisis in a legally and ethically appropriate manner. Because all team members are required to have a thorough understanding of the rules and regulations surrounding commitments, therapeutic holds, and procedural guidelines of relevant collateral agencies, this consultation should also serve to alert the supervisor to outside organizations (e.g., court, social service agency) that need to be involved in the treatment plan.

Finally, youth and family adherence to crisis treatment plans is essential in ensuring the safety of the client, family, therapist, and community. Thus, a critical element in MST crisis management is monitoring adherence to such plans through random spot checks in person or by phone; self-reports (e.g., from client, from caregivers); and reports of significant others involved in the crisis plan (e.g., siblings, extended family members, friends, neighbors).

## Crisis Plans

MST crisis plans should be based upon MST treatment principles and the philosophy of ecological validity. While some of principles may be more applicable than others during a given crisis, all MST crisis interventions should be based upon an accurate understanding of the fit of the current crisis (Principle 1) as developed during the crisis assessment detailed previously. In addition, the goals of the vast majority of crisis interventions should be designed to promote responsible behavior and decrease irresponsible behavior (Principle 3) by targeting well-defined and well-specified target behaviors (Principle 4). Thus, MST crisis plans typically incorporate behavioral interventions. In addition, crisis plans may integrate the use of psychopharmacological agents, especially when (1) the youth has a psychiatric condition such as ADHD or bipolar affective disorder in which medications have proven to be effective in treating symptoms (e.g., impulsivity, psychosis, mania) that are contributing to the current crisis, or (2) a youth's behavior is so extreme that he or she might inflict serious harm to self or others without psychopharmacological management.

### BEHAVIORAL INTERVENTIONS

Several behavioral interventions are routinely used in MST crisis plans. Choice of a behavioral intervention is based upon the function of the target behavior (e.g., suicidal threat, aggression). The function of the target behavior is determined through a functional analysis. The functional analysis serves as the basis for choosing among behavioral strategies (e.g., reinforcement, punishment, extinction), that is, interventions are logically based on the functional analysis.

A functional analysis focuses on three phases of behavior, the ABC's: (1) antecedents (e.g., triggers, situations, moods) or the context in which the behavior occurs (e.g., family fights when members are drinking), (2) behavior (e.g., aggression), and (3) consequences (e.g., reinforcement, punishment, extinction). A considerable amount of research has shown that events following behavior affect the future probability of the behavior. Events that increase behaviors are called *reinforcers*, and events that decrease behaviors are called *punishers*. If a pleasant event follows a particular behavior (e.g., withdrawal of aversive stimuli—demands are removed), the behavior is more probable in the future. Conversely, if an aversive event follows the behavior (e.g., extra chores), the behavior is less probable in the future. For example, a youth who responds to maternal requests with threats of physical aggression ("If you don't get out of my face, I'll punch you out!") is more likely to respond to future requests with similar behavior if the mother withdraws the request (the mother is negatively reinforcing verbal threats). Thus, behavior and events are functionally related—the function of the youth's threats of physical aggression was to terminate maternal requests for responsible behavior.

Withdrawal of reinforcement (i.e., extinction) causes an initial increase (i.e., extinction burst) and then a decrease in the targeted behavior (e.g., its intensity, its frequency, its duration). Thus, if the mother refused to back down from her demands, one would expect the youth's threatening behavior to escalate (extinction burst). This would constitute a "predictable crisis," as described previously, and the MST team would have to integrate a plan to treat this behavior into the larger Safety Plan.

Using the Safety Plan form (Figure 5.5), the crisis team members list in very clear language what will happen if the youth's behavior persists, escalates, or recurs. Behavioral interventions are listed from least aversive or intrusive to most aversive or restrictive. Care is taken to ensure that any intervention listed on the form has a reasonable chance of de-escalating the crisis or controlling the youth's behavior. An examination of the youth's previous history may provide this information. For example, if Johnny becomes angry and verbally threatens his family members, the first intervention may be that he is asked to take a time-out in his room by his mother. If he refuses and his agitation escalates and becomes potentially harmful, the second intervention may involve an assigned family or treatment team member therapeutically holding him, using the treatment team's approved protocol. If Johnny continues to be agitated and aggressive after 30 minutes, the next intervention may be to call police and have him taken to the local emergency room where he will be evaluated by the team psychiatrist. If his agitation continues in the emergency room, the final step may be to place him in a more restrictive setting such as a psychiatric hospital or detention. Note that care would be taken to use the least restrictive setting that is able to safely manage his symptoms.

Although MST crisis plans rely primarily upon psychosocial inter-

Safety Plan

The _____Family.

Criteria for Implementation of Crisis Plan (Be very specific):


Interventions (Least to most restrictive):


Medications:


Other:


**FIGURE 5.5.** MST Crisis Team Safety Plan Form.


ventions, such interventions may be insufficient when treating organically impaired youth (e.g., those with psychosis). Thus, when indicated, psychotropic medication protocols are integrated into MST Crisis Plans. Given that problem behavior is multidetermined, psychosocial interventions will nevertheless continue to be important for youth treated with medication. For example, a youth with bipolar affective disorder and symptoms of mania and agitation may demonstrate a large reduction in symptoms when receiving therapeutic doses of mood stabilizers. Psychosocial interventions to augment the pharmacological treatment may include educating the family about the illness and ways to detect early signs of relapse, behavioral interventions to manage behavior and increase medication compliance, and strategies to increase psychosocial supports.


PSYCHOPHARMACOLOGICAL INTERVENTIONS

Generally, the presence of the following three factors suggests the need for incorporating psychopharmacological interventions into the Safety Plan:

1. Escalating anger/aggression/psychosis despite behavioral interventions.
2. Difficulty complying with emergency treatment plans due to agitation, anger, or psychotic thoughts.
3. Need of rapid protection of the client and others from harm.

Before setting up a psychopharmacological intervention, the team psychiatrist must ensure that the youth is medically stable and obtain consent from the guardian and the youth. Currently, few uncontrolled studies (Joshi, Hamel, Joshi, & Capozzoli, 1998; Measham, 1995 ) and no controlled trials of medications for rapid stabilization of youth in psychiatric crisis have been conducted. However, trials have been conducted with adult populations (Resnick & Burton, 1984; Thomas, Schwartz, & Petrilli, 1992; Zealberg, Finkenbine, & Christie, 1995). Medications such as neuroleptics, lithium, antiepileptics, beta blockers, and alpha-adrenergic agonists have been used for the treatment of chronic behavioral disorders in adolescents (Green, 1995). Thus, the team's child psychiatrist must develop a drug administration protocol that is consistent with recent professional guidelines and local rules concerning dispensing and administering psychotropic medications in community-based clinic and emergency room settings.

## SPECIAL TOPICS

Treating youth experiencing a psychiatric emergency in the community poses many challenges that can be manageable with adequate training, forethought, and support. Foremost among the challenges is maintaining youth and family safety with a population of youth historically treated in restrictive settings.

### Use of Therapeutic Holds

On occasion, a youth's behavior is so extreme that therapeutic hold is required. When using therapeutic holds the emphasis should always be on the care, welfare, safety, and security of the client and those around him or her. Therapeutic hold is only recommended when the following criteria are met:

1. The team has received adequate training and certification in the use of therapeutic holds from the organization in which the team is housed.
2. The organization has established protocols for physical intervention with which team members are familiar.
3. The client presents a clear and present danger (e.g., the youth is homicidal, suicidal, or psychotic) to him- or herself or others.
4. Other techniques of behavioral control have been exhausted.
5. Supervisory permission, ideally from both the child psychiatrist and the MST supervisor, to hold the client has been obtained.

6. A minimum of two people are present. If adequate people are not present, the client should be allowed to leave and the police should be called (see police contact protocol) for immediate help.
7. The environment is free from sharp and other dangerous objects.

When these criteria are met and therapeutic holds are used, the following procedures should ensue. First, holds should never be employed for more than 30 minutes. If this maximum is exceeded, the client should be immediately transferred to a local emergency room (via EMS or police transport) where a psychiatric evaluation should be conducted (or the crisis treatment plan implemented, if one exists). Second, as suggested by Jacobs (1983), a debriefing period should follow the crisis in which the following questions are asked of those present: What were your reactions physically and emotionally? Could the situation have been handled differently? What worked well? What didn't work well? What seemed to happen right before this event that may have triggered or contributed to it? Finally, the reasons for using therapeutic holds must be clearly documented. In many settings, the team psychiatrist may be required to examine the youth and sign documents related to the therapeutic hold within a certain time period. MST teams must take care to follow the rules and regulations established by local, state, and federal professional regulatory agencies concerning therapeutic holds.

## Commitments

MST administrators and supervisors must have a thorough understanding of and familiarity with existing federal and state laws, and ethical guidelines surrounding commitments. This information should be shared with all members of the treatment team. Commitment laws vary from state to state, providing a wide range of standards and procedures for involuntary hospitalizations. Generally, however, two types of commitments are available in most localities: emergency and judicial. In an emergency commitment, a mental health professional (e.g., a psychiatrist) evaluates the client and determines that he or she poses a significant risk of harm to self or others due to mental illness and requires immediate psychiatric treatment. Paperwork (e.g., "commitment papers") is then completed and the client is immediately hospitalized. Judicial review will occur at some time interval after commitment, and a judge will sign an order to prolong the commitment if he or she feels this is indicated.

In a judicial commitment, family members or other laypeople may petition the court to involuntarily commit a person to treatment. A hearing is set and the court determines if the person poses a danger to self or others due to mental illness and requires involuntary placement in a treatment facility. As the laws and procedures concerning commitment vary from state to state, a protocol that is specific to the team's location should be developed by each MST team concerning how commitments will be handled. Note that all members of the MST team should understand how to conduct a commitment, but specific roles may be assigned to team members if indicated. For example, if a signature from a notary public is required to complete commitment papers, several team members (e.g., crisis caseworkers) may become notary publics to facilitate the commitment process when indicated.

## Police Interventions

Police often play important roles in MST crisis plans. For example, police have supported MST crisis plans via their physical presence, helped provide physical restraints, accompanied team members into volatile situations, and conducted drive-bys (i.e., "driving by" a home to see if things are okay). In addition, police have played an active role in crisis plans that require youth removal from a treatment site contingent upon aggression or threats of aggression. To obtain this level of cooperation with local police requires that team members follow several steps.

*First*, when communicating with the police (e.g., 911, dispatch officer, or other contact person), the nature of the request should be clarified (we need EMS, we need a police officer) and the role of the team member should be explained.

*Second*, upon the officer's arrival, the following steps should be followed.

1. A family member or treatment team member should be designated to meet the dispatched officer and ask for specific assistance.
2. The role of the MST team in crisis management should be explained, and a recommended intervention plan should be presented.
3. The team member should emphasize that the youth is already in outpatient treatment and that the officer's help is needed to provide safety and appropriate care for the youth and family.
4. Most importantly, the team member should emphasize that the MST team would like to continue to maintain responsibility for the client and the officer is seen as someone to assist in the crisis rather than as a solution to the crisis.

*Third*, the family, treatment team member, and police should agree upon an exact plan. The plan should include specific information concerning each person's role in the crisis plan and the conditions under which the plan will go into effect.

*Finally*, team and family members must treat the officer respectfully and remember that he or she is being asked to go out of his or her way to support the crisis plan. Thus, whenever possible, the officer should be thanked informally (e.g., with a thank you card) and formally (e.g., with a letter to the officer's supervisor).

## Professional Decorum

Since many youths served by the MST treatment team are likely to have multiple professionals representing a variety of agencies involved in their case, team members should cultivate positive relations with these individuals. Consistent with the MST approach to treating youths exhibiting serious antisocial behavior, team members should construct crisis plans involving other agencies in ways that minimize the work required of other professionals. Thus, the brunt of the work and responsibility for implementing crisis plans should rest with the family and the MST treatment team.

Each agency or professional group has a unique set of administrative protocols and procedures for interfacing with external entities. The following guidelines, drawn from the MST approach to school-based interventions, have been helpful in developing positive relationships between various professionals (e.g., teachers, case managers, other therapists) and families (these are described more extensively in Chapter 4):

1. Regular administrative channels at the agency should be followed before direct care professionals are contacted, and the administrative hierarchy should be honored. Consequently, the MST treatment team is responsible for "learning the ropes" of each agency.
2. When making a request or interacting with professionals, MST personnel should be nonthreatening and always convey respect for the professional.
3. MST personnel should arrange meetings or schedule appointments with professionals at a time and place convenient for the professionals.
4. During face-to-face meetings, MST personnel should emphasize respect for the professionals and their role in helping the youth, family, and treatment team.
5. Professionals should be thanked for their time and attention,

even if they contributed minimally to the development or implementation of the crisis plan. The liberal use of positive reinforcement can lead to better interpersonal relationships between the treatment team members and the professionals (or agencies), which increases the possibility that these individuals will contribute to current and future crisis plans.

Thus, having a comprehensive understanding of the context in which the MST treatment team is embedded is essential. This understanding and the ability to design and implement interventions based on the understanding will play a central role in facilitating outcomes for the families the team serves.

## CONCLUSION

MST crisis intervention strategies are founded on the premise that crises are often precipitated by a confluence of factors within the youth's social ecology, and importantly, each youth's presentation is individual and unique. Thus, safe and effective interventions can best be developed by first understanding the individual, family, peer, and community factors sustaining or diminishing the crisis. When this is understood, evidence-based effective interventions can be designed and implemented in ways that prioritize youth and community safety while promoting ecological validity.

# CHAPTER 6

# MST-Based Continuum of Care

This chapter describes an MST-based continuum of care designed to meet the chronic mental health needs of youths with serious emotional disturbance and their families. With home-based MST as its foundation, the continuum provides services ranging in intensity from outpatient care to psychiatric hospitalization. Importantly, no matter where the youth is placed in the continuum, the same therapist and psychiatrist provide treatment, and these professionals are working with the same MST supervisor. Hence, continuity of clinical decision making is high. Moreover, in contrast to traditional MST home-based services, treatment is not time-limited.

During the past decade, two limitations of the traditional MST approach to service delivery (i.e., 3–5 months of intensive home-based services and then treatment termination) have become apparent. First, in light of the substantive and serious clinical challenges presented by youths at imminent risk of out-of-home placement and their families, many families require services beyond the 3- to 5-month limit of MST programs. Faced with continued clinical need, traditional MST programs have tried to refer such children and their families to those community resources that best match their clinical needs and use evidence-based treatments. Unfortunately, few community programs use evidence-based practices, and these programs rarely have the financial and training resources needed to overcome barriers to service access and implement the strong quality assurance mechanisms needed to attain desired clinical outcomes. Hence, effective follow-through on the continued clinical needs of children and families is unfortunately infrequent.

A second limitation of traditional MST programs has been their relative inability to influence treatment decisions following crises that require placement of the youth outside the family. For example, the youth might present suicidal behavior that leads to emergency psychiatric hospitalization, or the adolescent might commit a criminal offense that leads juvenile justice authorities to place him or her in a residential treatment center. In both instances, clinical decision-making authority is taken away from the MST program, the youth is removed from his or her natural environment, services are provided that likely have little to do with learning how to function effectively in noninstitutional settings (e.g., milieu therapy in the hospital, positive peer culture group treatment in the residential facility), evidence-based treatments are infrequently used, and few resources are devoted to improving the capacity of the youth's caregivers to meet his or her mental health needs (Barker, 1998; Joshi & Rosenberg, 1997; U.S. Public Health Service, 2000). These limitations have clearly restricted the ability of MST to achieve desired outcomes (i.e., improved functioning and reduced placements) in the indicated cases.

The significance of these limitations has been further reinforced by our experience in conducting the randomized trial of MST as an alternative to the psychiatric hospitalization of youths presenting mental health emergencies (Henggeler, Rowland, et al., 1997, 1999). The chronicity of the youth and family mental health problems was difficult to address with a treatment duration limited to approximately 4 months. On the other hand, progress was made in designing MST-compatible placements—that is, placements where the MST psychiatrist and team controlled clinical decision making, including the timing of admission and discharge, and delivered the clinical services. As discussed later in this chapter, the nature of the clinical services provided to youths in MST-controlled placements and their families differ substantially from those provided to other youths in those placements.

Fortuitously, the emerging success of the alternative to hospitalization project (Henggeler, Rowland, et al., 1999; Schoenwald, Ward, Henggeler, & Rowland, 2000) coincided with a request from a major foundation to help move evidence-based mental health practices for economically disadvantaged children and their families into urban settings. Dr. Patrick McCarthy, director of policy reform and initiative management for the Annie E. Casey Foundation, approached the Family Services Research Center (FSRC) with an invitation to collaborate in moving evidence-based practices into the sites of the foundation's Mental Health Initiative for Urban Children. Essentially, the leadership at the foundation were drawing the same conclusions that others (e.g., Burns et al., 1999; Henggeler, Schoenwald, & Munger, 1996; Weisz, Han, & Valeri, 1997) were reaching about the advantages and limitations of system reform with regard to clinical outcomes for children. That is, while system reform can improve service-level outcomes (Bickman, Noser, & Summerfelt, 1999; Bickman, Summerfelt, & Noser, 1997), the key to improving clinical-level outcomes is the provision of treatments with known efficacy (i.e., evidence-based services; see Weisz & Jensen, 1999).

In light of the commitment of the FSRC to rigorous evaluation and our view that the field would be well served by the validation of an evidence-based continuum of care, we agreed to collaborate in the development and testing of an MST continuum in at least two sites. The Annie E. Casey Foundation funded the development of treatment manuals for the components of the continuum of care, supported the recruitment of collaborating sites, is supporting the research of the randomized trials of the continua, and is funding much of the training and ongoing quality assurance needed to maintain treatment fidelity in the continuum. As discussed in Chapter 8, the Philadelphia site began recruitment of youth and families in June 2001.

The MST continua focus on those youths who are presenting the most complex and costly clinical problems in the community or state. The fundamental purpose of the MST continuum is to provide high-quality evidence-based services that follow the youth at all points of the continuum and are sustained for as long as required to maintain favorable outcomes. Thus, the MST-based continuum of care is a clinically integrated system of mental health and substance abuse services for youth experiencing serious clinical problems in which all practitioners implement and adhere to the principles and techniques of multisystemic therapy. The MST-based continuum of care includes full-time clinicians dedicated solely to the provision of MST services. The following mental health and substance abuse service delivery mechanisms are part of the MST continuum: home-based services, intensive outpatient services, crisis intervention, family resource specialists/parent partners, therapeutic foster care, respite services, and access to residential and hospital beds. The organizational chart for the MST continuum in Philadelphia is provided in Figure 6.1 as an example.

As depicted in Figure 6.1, a central and critical feature of the MST continuum is that *no matter where the youth is placed in the continuum, treatment is provided by the same therapist and psychiatrist, and these*

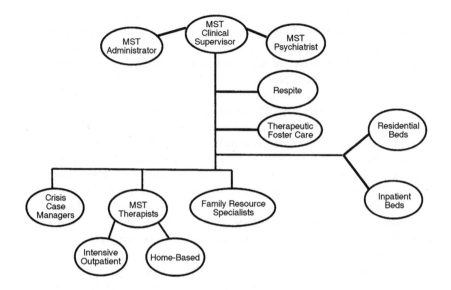

**FIGURE 6.1.** Philadelphia MST continuum of care.

*professionals are working with the same MST supervisor.* Moreover, each of these professionals is operating from the same evidence-based perspective and working within intensive quality assurance protocols. Thus, continuity of clinical decision making is extremely high.

The MST continuum includes several models of service delivery. The features of MST using the home-based model of service delivery have been described previously. Intensive outpatient MST is essentially the same approach with a higher caseload (e.g., 10 families per therapist). Intensive outpatient MST is intended for youths and families who no longer require the intensity of home-based services, but still have a substantive need for mental health services to maintain functioning and reduce the probability of out-of-home placements. Intensive outpatient care is a "low-dose" model of MST treatment, rather than the array of services typically found in outpatient clinics (e.g., individual treatment, group treatment, diagnostic assessments). That is, the master's-level clinician, located in the MST site in a community setting, conducts assessments and interventions in accordance with MST principles, but sessions are held less frequently than in MST home-based services. Though based in a community location, the MST intensive outpatient clinician also meets with families in their homes and in schools as needed.

The remainder of this chapter describes those service components that are critical to the MST continuum and that have not been described previously. These include the integration of family resource specialists into MST teams; the use of respite care, foster care, and residential/hospital services; and the integration of psychopharmacological treatment.

## ROLE OF THE FAMILY RESOURCE
## SPECIALIST IN THE MST TREATMENT TEAM

Family resource specialists (FRS) are full-time high school- or college-graduate level members of the MST team who ideally reside in the neighborhoods most frequently served by the MST continuum. The FRS assist the MST clinical team with functions in five important areas: (1) cultural competence, (2) engagement, (3) assessment, (4) intervention, and (5) overcoming barriers to treatment. To function effectively in these areas, the FRS must have in-depth knowledge of the community in which they work. For example, the FRS should know if certain houses shelter criminal activity or if drug deals frequently occur in certain locations or at certain times. The FRS should also have a sense of who the community leaders are and what prosocial activities or resources are available for family members. Likewise, the FRS must develop a complete understanding of the clinical team's perspective and keep all information obtained while working with family members confidential. Participation in clinical supervisory sessions is essential for FRS. Like all members of the MST clinical team, the FRS only provides services that have been approved by the MST supervisor and that target the overarching goals of the treatment plan.

### Enhancing Cultural Competence

The FRS should have a good working knowledge of the community in which the family resides. This includes being familiar with the various cultures, traditions, and beliefs held by residents of the neighborhood. This knowledge will allow the FRS to give meaningful input into therapeutic decisions made by the clinical team and thereby increase the chances that interventions will be culturally appropriate and sensitive to the needs of the family and its surrounding neighborhood.

For example, an MST therapist working with a family was having great difficulty engaging the father in treatment. She had attempted to meet the father on several occasions, but because he was often away working, she met with the youth's mother and proceeded with an intervention to get a behavioral plan in place for the youth. The mother was unable to implement the plan, however. A significant barrier seemed to be the lack of buy-in from the father. The therapist had asked the mother to have the father call her to schedule an appointment, but this engagement strategy was not successful. The FRS helped the therapist develop more successful strategies for meeting the father by pointing out that in the family's culture, the father was responsible for making all decisions concerning the moral development and behavioral management of the children. Thus, the therapist had inadvertently violated a cultural rule by enlisting the mother to develop a behavioral plan without first obtaining the father's consent. Subsequently, the FRS worked with the therapist to help develop strategies to meet with and engage the father.

## Facilitating Engagement

FRS knowledge and understanding of the community and its residents may greatly help the treatment team engage the family in treatment. The FRS should strive to understand both the goals of the family and the perspective of the clinical team. The FRS can then problem-solve with team members when barriers to engagement arise. Initially, team members may have to rely on FRS to help engage families. As the therapists establish their own credibility and develop trustworthy interactions with the family, they should need less help from the FRS.

Here is an example of how the FRS can facilitate engagement. A therapist was having a very difficult time engaging a family in treatment. When he spoke with the family on the telephone they were receptive and seemed interested in treatment. Yet when he visited the house to meet the family, they would not even come to the door. The FRS was from the neighborhood and had no difficulty gaining admittance to the home. Further assessment of the situation by the FRS revealed that the family was not meeting with the therapist due to fear: they were afraid that drug dealers in the community would think that the therapist was a plain-clothes police detective and retaliate against the family. This was a reasonable fear given the high crime rate in the neighborhood and anticrime initiatives then underway by the local police. Hence, a plan was developed in which the therapist wore a white lab coat to the house, and the family and FRS spread the word throughout the community that the family was receiving medical care from a visiting nurse specialist.

## Helping with Assessments

Clinical assessments occur on an ongoing basis for each family receiving MST. The FRS may be asked to help with an assessment by observing family members and providing feedback to support or refute the team's clinical hypotheses. For example, a FRS might be assigned to drive a mother to the grocery store. The FRS might be asked to observe the mother interact with her children in the store and to note the strategies she used to get each to comply with her directives.

The therapist, however, must make sure that the FRS is fully educated concerning the assignment. In the previous example, the FRS should understand why the team wants to know about discipline strategies, how this information is assisting the team's understanding of the fit of the targeted problems, and how to formulate his or her response. Thus, the therapist may need to review the "fit circles" currently in place for the family and then provide the FRS with information about parenting styles, how to conceptualize certain parent–child interactions, and the team's hypotheses concerning what types of parenting styles the mother might demonstrate and how the assessment information will facilitate the attainment of overarching goals.

The FRS might also independently make observations that assist the clinical team with their ongoing assessment. For example, the FRS might meet a friend or sibling of the caregiver who is able to play a supportive role in treatment, yet has not been identified by the therapist. Again, it is imperative that the FRS become an integral part of the treatment team, with a working knowledge of the fit circles, overarching goals, and logic of interventions designed to reach these goals for each family served.

## Working with Therapists to Implement Interventions

The FRS also helps in implementing interventions. The therapist assigned to the family is responsible for ensuring that the FRS is given adequate training and resources to perform interventions and monitor outcomes. For example, a therapist was helping a teacher develop a behavioral program for an MST youth in her classroom. After monitoring this process for several days, the therapist found that the teacher seemed to be implementing the plan fairly well, but continued to need some assistance to ensure that consequences were applied consistently. With the supervisor's involvement, the therapist explained the behavioral plan to the FRS and gave him specific instructions on how to intervene if certain predictable situations occurred. The therapist was available to the FRS by cell phone, and provided daily follow-up to ensure that the interventions were effective.

While FRS may help therapists deliver a wide variety of treatments, one frequently used intervention that fits the role of the FRS particularly well is that of increasing indigenous social support.

## IMPORTANCE OF SOCIAL SUPPORT

Some families served by MST programs have very few social supports and are socially isolated. This isolation is a significant risk factor for a host of psychosocial problems, including domestic violence, child abuse and neglect, and mental illness (House, Landis, & Umberson, 1988). Social isolation serves as an obstacle to the acquisition and implementation of parenting skills (Baker, 1983; Wahler, 1980), and can attenuate treatment generalization and the maintenance of therapeutic gains (Wahler, 1990). Thus, assistance from social support networks is of critical importance in ensuring that families have the resources to nurture healthy development in their children. FRS may be asked to help expand and diversify a family's social network.

Since one of the goals of MST is to help families make changes that can be sustained (i.e., generalization), interventions involving social support systems should strive to tap the most proximal means of social support available. Thus, family members, friends, and neighbors should be targeted to fulfill social support functions before accessing more formal resources such as community or state agencies. Utilizing informal social supports has five distinct advantages. First, informal supports are more likely to meet the family's immediate needs. For example, informal supports are often more successful than formal sources such as employment agencies in helping unemployed persons find jobs (Athanasou, 1994; Rife & Belcher, 1994). Second, informal supports are more likely to provide resources that are timely and easily accessible (Henggeler et al., 1998). Third, informal supports are more likely to be sustained following treatment termination, as neighbors continue to be neighbors and friends continue to be friends. Fourth, informal supports are more likely to facilitate adherence to treatment regimens (Meichenbaum & Turk, 1987) through their acknowledgment and praise of newfound behavioral changes (i.e., positive reinforcement of adaptive behavior). Fifth, the reciprocity required to obtain informal supports (i.e., customary give-and-take) is more likely than formal supports to bolster a person's confidence and sense of self-sufficiency, which are prerequisites for empowerment.

When assessments performed by MST clinicians indicate that the lack of appropriate social supports is a factor that contributes significantly to the identified problems, increasing social support may become a treatment goal. When this goal has been set, the MST supervisor and clinical team can decide how to best intervene. These interventions frequently involve FRS.

## HELPING FAMILIES TO TAP SOCIAL SUPPORT RESOURCES

MST focuses on developing an ecologically based continuum of social supports for families ranging from friends, neighbors, and coworkers to civic and religious organizations to business and government agencies. A skilled and knowledgeable FRS can facilitate the use of multiple components of this continuum to help families expand and diversify their social support network. FRS may help families to tap social support resources through two processes: (1) increasing a family member's opportunities to meet prosocial supportive individuals, and (2) teaching parents requisite interpersonal skills (based on community norms) to access and/or take advantage of opportunities to gain support. Regarding the former process, the FRS might help parents meet potential sources of social support in the community through (1) community meetings (e.g., neighborhood watch, tenant associations), (2) community activities (e.g., cultural events, church activities), or (3) personal introductions (e.g., arranging meetings with indigenous leaders in the community). Generally, FRS can help parents become active participants in community activities that are likely to expand and diversify the pool of eligible social supports for a family. Regarding the latter process, building sustainable relationships is never easy, particularly if one does not have the requisite interpersonal skills. If the clinical team's assessment identifies lack of interpersonal skills as a barrier to obtaining social support, the FRS may be asked to help parents develop skills through social skills training, including the use of modeling and constructive feedback. Importantly, social skills taught by a competent person from the social community of which a parent is a part (e.g., FRS) are more likely to meet the sociocultural norms and context of that community than social skills taught by someone from outside the community (for a discussion, see Kazdin, 1982).

## Identifying and Overcoming Barriers to Treatment

The MST therapist is responsible for monitoring the outcome of therapeutic interventions and determining what barriers may be attenuating success. The FRS might be asked by the clinical team to aid in this process or might make independent observations that prove useful for the clinical team. For example, the FRS working with a family might have insights concerning why a family is having problems interfacing with school personnel that are based in cultural or community norms that the therapist does not recognize. Again, the FRS must have a good understanding of the fit circles and overarching and intermediary goals in place for a family to best assist with their treatment.

## Summary

By serving as a linkage between families, the community, and the MST continuum team, the FRS can enhance the team's cultural competence and help link families with ecologically valid social support systems. FRS also play an integral role in delivering MST by assisting therapists with assessments and interventions. Because FRS are members of the clinical team, they must maintain an understanding of the always evolving MST clinical picture and treatment plans in place for the families they serve. Like all members of the clinical team, the FRS only provide services that target the overarching goals of the MST treatment plan and that have been approved by the MST supervisor.

## RESPITE CARE

Most of what has been written about respite care services can be found in the developmental disabilities and mental retardation literatures. Although there is no consensus on a definition of respite care in these literatures, *respite care* is commonly described as intermittent care provided for the families of developmentally disabled individuals living at home for the purpose of providing an interval of relief to caregivers from the physical and emotional demands of caregiving (Joyce & Singer, 1983; Upshur, 1982a, 1982b; Warren & Cohen, 1985). Within this context, respite care is used during emergencies, to provide parents and family members relief from the day-to-day responsibilities of caring for someone with significant developmental delays, to allow time for individual and/or family development, to allow time for more mundane purposes such as running errands or keeping appointments, or when families are taking a vacation. The underlying rationale of respite care is to provide families a period for relief and revitalization, and to prevent (or delay) family breakdown and institutionalization of the children (Halpern, 1985). Studies in the field of developmental disabilities suggest that respite care can improve family functioning (Cohen, 1982; Joyce & Singer, 1983), reduce stress (Apolloni & Triest, 1983), enhance the coping resources of mothers (Rimmerman, Krammer, Levy, & Levy, 1989), and decrease the placement of children in out-of-home care (Cohen, 1982; Salisbury & Intagliata, 1986; Upshur, 1982a, 1982b). Research specifically on respite care used by families of youth with serious behavioral and emotional problems is insufficient to draw any conclusions on the effectiveness of the service (Boothroyd, Kuppinger, Evans, Armstrong, & Radigan, 1998). Nevertheless, respite care is increasingly a topic of discussion among caregivers and service providers.

### Objective of Respite in an MST-Based Continuum of Care

MST respite is only used in the service of a treatment goal. Common goals of MST-based respite include engaging families in treatment, conducting assessments, implementing interventions, and overcoming treatment barriers. Thus, in contrast with some respite programs that provide youth with a variety of activities and events not ordinarily available to them (e.g., trips to the zoo, camps that families couldn't ordinarily afford), MST-based respite is focused, often brief, and designed to facilitate the youth's continued participation in his or her daily activities (e.g., school, extracurricular activities, contact with prosocial peers). From a MST perspective, the family, not the treatment team, is ultimately responsible for exposing children to activities that promote positive development. When financial constraints present barriers to doing this, families learn to marshal resources in a variety of ways, including applying for scholarships to participate in scout or sports activities, seeking no-cost options at church or community recreation centers, and participating in school- or church-sponsored fund drives for special trips.

Because MST-based respite is a service rather than a placement, it can be provided anywhere, to anyone in the youth's ecology, for varying lengths of time. Possible locations in which respite may occur include a family's home, the community, or a respite care provider's home. The duration of respite can vary from a few hours to several days. In a range from informal to formal supports, respite may be provided by individuals in the family's natural environment (e.g., neighbors, extended family), any member of the treatment team, or individuals employed by the team specifically to provide respite. Respite funds can also be used (preferentially) to pay people in the natural ecology (e.g., relatives, neighbors) to perform respite tasks. Respite services by formal service providers, however, should be used only when the indigenous or proximal resources are not available. The *nature* of the respite activity may vary from watching a mother's children while she purchases groceries to staying in a family's home overnight to help monitor an agitated youth. The provider of respite care works with the child, caregiver, or individuals in the school or community to meet the overarching goals targeted by the respite intervention.

The number of times a family can use respite services is not limited. Repeated use, however, may indicate that the MST treatment plan needs to be reconfigured to better address the precipitants of requests for respite and the natural ecology's ability to support the family. Per usual, all respite interventions should be based on the MST conceptualization of the fit of identified problems and carried out in the service of overarching treatment goals with the approval of the MST supervisor.

## Examples of Appropriate Uses of MST-Based Respite

The key question when deciding whether or not to use MST respite is, "Is respite in the service of a specific treatment goal?" Respite should always be designed to facilitate the attainment of a specific treatment goal.

Two conclusions follow from this assertion. First, using respite just because it is available is inappropriate. Second, given that treatment goals are individualized for each family, a respite service (e.g., babysitting) that may be appropriate in one family context may be inappropriate in another family context. The following examples illustrate appropriate uses of respite.

## PROMOTING ENGAGEMENT

*Engagement* is the process by which the therapist connects with the caregiver and builds a collaborative working relationship. *A collaborative working relationship* means that therapists and caregivers make therapeutic decisions jointly, and that caregivers are treated as important members of the treatment team. Engagement includes understanding the caregiver's world, the problems that have resulted in the referral to treatment, and the caregiver's goals, hopes, and desires. Moreover, the process of engagement must be sustained throughout treatment and is characterized by empathy, responsiveness, warmth, concerned involvement, and respect (Cunningham & Henggeler, 1999).

Although the MST therapist is responsible for designing and helping the family implement strategies to effectively meet treatment goals, sometimes a caregiver is too exhausted or frustrated to free up the emotional or mental energy needed to participate in treatment. The therapist, consequently, may decide that a break from childcare responsibilities would facilitate engagement. In such a case, the therapist and the family would first seek out individuals in the caregiver's support system willing to care for the children for the day. If the therapist–family team is unable to cultivate such support, or the available support is unable to meet the imminent need, MST-based respite services could be provided. In the interest of engagement, treatment would initially focus on goals that were important to the caregiver—even if these were not directly connected to the ultimate goals of stakeholders. By focusing on the needs of the *person*, not just the *person-as-parent*, the therapist can often facilitate the engagement process.

## AIDING ASSESSMENT

Obtaining a comprehensive assessment of the factors driving and sustaining youth behavior provides the foundation for development of appropriate interventions. Accurate understanding of such behavior is facilitated by observing the youth and individuals in the youth's ecology across multiple contexts. At times, respite care providers may be given the assignment of helping the clinical team assess a situation. For instance, a neighbor, who is paid respite funds to monitor a MST youth and her siblings after school each day, may be asked to note the number of verbally aggressive statements the youth makes to her siblings and to determine if various sibling or care provider responses increase or decrease this behavior. Respite providers who assist with monitoring youth in school may track how the behavior of the teacher and peers in the classroom affects the client's behaviors.

## FACILITATING INTERVENTIONS

Respite care providers often implement clinical interventions with the guidance of the therapist and the clinical team. For example, a family member who is paid respite funds to assist the parents in supervising a youth will be expected to carefully implement the behavioral plans developed by the family and treatment team. Respite care workers may also follow protocols to prompt youth they are supervising in social skills or to assist caregivers or teachers in implementing interventions.

## ADDRESSING TREATMENT BARRIERS

Barriers to change often arise during the course of treatment. The clinical team is responsible for designing and implementing interventions to overcome such barriers. For example, Jason's relationships with deviant peers and the lack of structured well-supervised time after school were significant drivers of Jason's antisocial behavior. Leveraging his strengths— athletic ability and interest in sports—the therapist and his mother helped Jason join the high school football team as an intervention to increase his structured time with prosocial peers and promote school involvement. This strategy worked well for several weeks until the family car was stolen. Since the family lived 10 miles from the school and could not afford to replace the vehicle, transportation became a significant barrier to Jason's continued involvement in football. Initially, since the mother could not muster the support to provide this service, she was planning to take Jason out of football. The therapist, consequently, enlisted respite care workers to provide transportation until she could help the mother develop a more ecological alternative. Ultimately, Jason was able to work out an agreement with an elderly neighbor in which he cared for her yard in return for rides home from practice.

## Key Elements of MST-Based Respite Care

### RESPITE CARE PROVIDERS

As noted previously, respite can be provided by members of the treatment team (e.g., FRS, crisis caseworkers, therapists) as well as by indigenous supports (e.g., extended family, friends, neighbors) and professionals (e.g., foster parents). Irrespective of which source of respite is used, providers must have a commitment to helping children, be willing and able to collaborate with the MST therapist and caregivers, and have the ability to maintain a safe and nurturing environment while a youth is in their care. For reasons of ecological validity, sustainability, and caregivers' comfort about entrusting the safety of their children to others, respite care providers should first be recruited from among relatives, family friends, and neighbors. Similarly, the same respite care provider should be linked with the family whenever possible. Consistent with this perspective, research has shown that family members are more likely to use and benefit from respite when they trust and feel comfortable with the respite care provider (Boothroyd et al., 1998). Although family comfort level is an important factor in selecting respite providers, the primary consideration remains the provider's capacity to facilitate the goals of the respite service.

## THERAPIST RESPONSIBILITIES

The MST therapist, in collaboration with the caregiver, is responsible for delineating the functions of respite and for optimizing its utility. Hence, the therapist monitors the use of respite and ensures that the goals and objectives of respite—engagement, assessment, intervention, addressing treatment barriers—are actually met. For example, if respite is used to give a single father a break from caring for several young children so that the therapist can more easily engage him in the treatment of his adolescent son, the therapist should actively work to align with the father while the children are receiving respite care. If the therapist simply leaves the father alone to rest from childrearing stresses while the children are away, the use of respite is not appropriate because progress toward treatment goals is not being made. The following case illustrates the multiple tasks the therapist must perform to ensure that respite is used effectively. In this example, respite was used to help overcome significant treatment barriers.

The Jones family is headed by a single mother who works a minimum-wage job and is raising four children between the ages of 4 and 15 years in a two-bedroom apartment in a subsidized housing project in a high-crime neighborhood. Ms. Jones's relatives live in another state, as does her ex-husband, who has not paid child support for several years. Her 15-year-old son, Markus, had been placed in various residential settings since the age of 10 years due to his persistent physical aggression at school and in the home, criminal activities, and substance use. When Ms. Jones and the MST therapist began to implement an intensive monitoring plan for Markus, he became increasingly agitated and verbally abusive. Concomitantly, Ms. Jones became increasingly fatigued and depressed about her life, complaining that she had no one to turn to for support and could see no end to her problems.

One of the initial goals of treatment was to develop more effective monitoring and supervision of Markus's activities. In light of Ms. Jones's work schedule, the absence of extended family in the community, and her social isolation, indigenous supports needed to be developed to facilitate the goal of providing increased monitoring of Markus. Hence, a decision was made to identify neighbors who could assist Ms. Jones in monitoring Markus after school. Barriers to implementing this plan, however, included Ms. Jones's work hours, her fatigue, and her reluctance to "air dirty laundry" with neighbors she barely knew or to trust neighbors who themselves might be using drugs. To address these barriers, the therapist reframed "airing dirty laundry" as solicitation of needed support, helped identify which neighbors did not use drugs and were acceptable to Ms. Jones, and implemented cognitive-behavioral strategies to address her depressive thoughts. By the end of the week, however, Ms. Jones remained too disheartened to use the cognitive-behavioral strategies, engage neighbors, or exert the necessary effort to implement the monitoring plan, which precipitated threats of violence from Markus. Thus, Markus remained involved with gang-affiliated peers, continued using marijuana, and thereby violated the terms of his probation. At this juncture, the therapist and Ms. Jones determined that respite might be useful in eliminating treatment barriers that had surfaced (i.e., the feelings of fatigue and depression, the lack of contact with neighbors, and the backlash from Markus). The working hypothesis was that respite would help Ms. Jones get some rest, which, in combination with therapist efforts, would help her feel less depressed about her life and better able to stand fast with Markus.

Formal respite care was arranged to begin Friday after school and end Sunday afternoon, as Ms. Jones had Saturday off work. Because the respite caregiver, a foster parent, was not familiar to Ms. Jones or the children, the therapist arranged for all parties to meet on Thursday evening. In light of Markus's aggressive behavior and association with deviant peers, the therapist stayed with the respite caregiver when rules were described and then spent several hours at the caregiver's home on Friday evening to ensure that monitoring of Markus was sufficient. The therapist also drove by the respite provider's home twice on Saturday to facilitate adherence to the behavioral plan. On Sunday, the therapist and Ms. Jones met for 3 hours before the children returned to consider the fit of Ms. Jones's fatigue that contributed to the need for respite and to alter the MST treatment plan to more quickly and comprehensively address the variety of circumstances that led to the use of formal respite. To this end, the therapist asked Ms. Jones's permission to seek other community-based sources of support. The therapist also volunteered to be at the Jones's home for an hour before school and after school and at the time of Markus's appointed curfew to assist Ms. Jones with managing the needs of all four children at these high-risk times (i.e., these times are when sibling altercations and conflict between Ms. Jones and Markus often occurred). In addition, Ms. Jones and the therapist sought tempo-rary monitoring assistance from Markus's probation officer. Thus, be-fore the respite period ended, a plan was in place whereby Ms. Jones knew she would have additional assistance to help combat the cumula-tive effects of daily stressors until neighbors or acquaintances from church could be contacted and engaged to provide such assistance.

## THERAPEUTIC FOSTER CARE

The primary goal of therapeutic foster care (TFC) within the MST continuum is to provide an opportunity to alter the environment of the family of origin to safely support their child in their home. Foster care placement, therefore, is viewed as an intervention to support parents/ caregivers, not as a child intervention. Children are not placed in foster care as a result of their own psychological or behavioral problems; rather, they are placed because of the inability of their environment to safely and effectively meet their needs. While traditional foster care typi-cally views parents whose children are placed in foster care as being "un-fit," MST views most such caregivers as capable of being effective if pro-vided with treatment that targets the multiple factors that compromised their ability to care for their children. Indeed, recent research supports this perspective, suggesting that when children at risk of placement are allowed to remain at home and biological families are given the re-sources typically given to foster families (e.g., training, treatment, money, respite), biological families are able to achieve the same or better outcomes with their children as are foster parents (Evans, Armstrong, & Kuppinger, 1996).

### Pathways between MST Home-Based Care and TFC

The ultimate goal of MST is to empower families to keep their children at home, in school, and out of trouble. When circumstances in the home environment render placement with the family, relatives, or friends un-safe or untenable, TFC is often the placement of choice because it pro-vides the least restrictive living environment.

## FROM HOME-BASED TO TFC

Youth receiving home-based MST are generally placed in foster care via two pathways. On the first path, which is most commonly used by current service systems, the team concludes that the youth is in significant danger of abuse or neglect and needs to be removed from the home to ensure his or her safety. Thus, while MST puts a premium on treating youth in their natural ecology, family unification is not prioritized over the safety of the youth and family members. If abuse or neglect is occurring and presents significant concern for safety, the appropriate social service authorities are informed, as required by state and federal law. The therapist then works with the social service agency and the family to develop the most appropriate placement plan for the youth. When adequate indigenous placement sources are not available, the treatment team will attempt to access a TFC placement within the MST continuum.

On the second path, with the caregiver's consent, the treatment team may place the youth in foster care in the service of treatment goals. These placements may be short term (e.g., 1–30 days), and conceptualized as a type of respite, or of longer duration (e.g., 1–6 months), and thus more appropriately conceptualized as foster care. When used in the service of treatment goals, as described subsequently, TFC, like respite, can facilitate attainment of goals related to engagement, assessment, intervention design, or treatment barriers. Placement into TFC, therefore, should not be considered as an indication of treatment failure. Rather, TFC becomes yet another tool in the team's repertoire for designing effective interventions.

## FROM TFC TO FAMILY OF ORIGIN

Some youth entering MST treatment may already be living with foster families. Among these, some may be considered permanent foster placements while others may be eligible for reunification with family members. Because individuals usually remain connected with family throughout their lifespan, and service systems often fail to provide adequate stability in the lives of youth in foster placement (McDonald, Allen, Westerfelt, & Piliavin, 1996), the MST team expends extraordinary effort in locating a caregiver in the natural ecology (i.e., family of origin and extended family) to parent the youth. In some cases, such resources may not exist (e.g., father deceased, mother in prison, no known relatives). For these adolescents, after making certain that more ecological supports are truly unavailable, the treatment team usually focuses on developing the foster parents' ability to care for the youth. Once the youth is stabilized in the foster home, the team works to solidify the foster family's relationship with the youth. Permanency planning (i.e., adoption, a long-term agreement with a social service agency concerning placement), if clinically appropriate, will be used to promote stability and to facilitate the maintenance of treatment gains. On the other hand, when a potentially viable caregiver in the natural ecology is identified, the MST therapist assesses and works with this caregiver (e.g., parents, stepparents, aunts, uncles, older siblings, grandparents) as well as with the foster family, striving to transition the youth back to family members safely.

## Tasks to Be Accomplished during Foster Care Placement

Several tasks must be accomplished by the MST team during a foster placement. The overriding purposes of these tasks are to minimize disruption of the youth's life and to optimize the likelihood of successful reunification.

### SAFETY

The therapist's first task is to strive for adequate resolution of the factors that resulted in the out-of-home placement. Behavior that threatens the safety of self or others is addressed in much the same way as any referral behavior (e.g., stealing cars, running away), except that a higher level of urgency is placed on ensuring that interventions are carried out with integrity and plans (safety plans) are implemented that adequately monitor and provide for quick corrections of the behavior of concern. Thus, when MST therapists are treating families whose children have been placed in a foster home, with or without the team's involvement, for issues concerning safety, abuse, or neglect, several tasks must be accomplished. Therapists must develop an understanding of the fit of the youth and family member transactions that resulted in placement. Then, following the MST treatment process outlined in Chapter 2, therapists work with supervisors to develop treatment strategies targeting the sequences of behavior that gave rise to the out-of-home placement.

### AGREEING ON GOALS OF PLACEMENT

Second, therapists must ensure that all stakeholders have a shared understanding of the measurable outcomes to be attained with placement. Foster care in the MST continuum will, by definition, involve at least four entities: the family of origin, the foster family, the MST treatment team, and the agency in which foster care is housed (if it is not part of the same agency as the MST treatment team). Often, the department of social services and other systems with legal mandates are also involved.

Hence, to facilitate the overarching goals of treatment, these entities must be in consensus regarding the measurable outcomes that will be achieved prior to the child's return home. The MST therapist, with help from the MST supervisor and other team members, must work with each stakeholder to gain buy-in for MST treatment goals, ensure ongoing adequate communication, and resolve barriers that may arise and threaten outcomes.

## COORDINATING TREATMENT ACROSS SYSTEMS

A third mission of therapists treating youth in foster care is the coordination of treatment across the family of origin and foster family. Because MST strives to promote treatment generalization and the long-term maintenance of therapeutic change (Principle 9), therapists must take care to ensure that interventions leverage the strengths of both families and increase the likelihood that the family of origin will be able to maintain therapeutic gains. Thus, therapists assess the strengths and needs in the ecologies of the foster family and the family of origin, strive to coordinate interventions between both families to create consistency across home environments, and plan for ways to generalize the gains made in the foster home back into the family of origin. Likewise, interventions in the foster home can be modified based on their successful implementation in the natural ecology (e.g., school, community recreation center).

## PROMOTING STABILITY

Fourth, therapists working with foster families should always strive to preserve the youth's natural ecology. To promote treatment generalization and minimize disruptive change in the life of the youth, the team should make every attempt (unless prohibited for safety reasons) to maintain the youth's connections to the community in which his or her family of origin resides. Thus, a high priority is placed on finding foster families that are part of the youth's community. Care is taken to ensure that the youth continues to attend the same school and continues to participate in prosocial activities with appropriate peers and family members. While preserving this continuity in the youth's life might require considerable logistical resources (e.g., transporting the youth to school and soccer games) and be inconvenient to providers, such expenditures are clearly in the youth's and the family's best long-term interest.

## VISITATION

When the factors driving the lack of safety in the family of origin have been identified and interventions have been put into place to make the changes needed to support the youth safely in the home, youth and family visitation are encouraged. Prior to visitation, however, the MST team must ensure that a safety plan is in place and will be appropriately implemented. The safety plan stems from a thorough assessment and understanding (i.e., functional analysis) of the events that set off or predispose the family to safety risk and the events that facilitate or inhibit the behaviors of concern. A well-developed safety plan should specify the rules the parents and youth must follow to reduce risk and outline the changes the youth and family members will make to support safety of the child. Importantly, a responsible family member who has the requisite emotional and mental stability needed to ensure implementation of the safety plan (see Chapter 5) should be identified and appropriately utilized in the plan. Given that caregivers whose children have been removed for safety reasons may not easily be able to assume full responsibility for their child's safety, the initial plan often uses indigenous family supports or more formal services such as MST clinicians or respite providers. Thus, the therapist may be involved with the family during initial visitations and provide periodic check-ins as the family demonstrates the ability to safely implement the plan.

## REUNIFICATION

An overarching goal of MST is to have youth live in the least restrictive setting that is feasible with a permanent caregiver who is able to provide appropriate levels of nurturance, support, and discipline. Hence, MST therapists generally strive to reunify youth and family members as soon as safely possible. This is done when risk factors that contributed to safety concerns have been significantly impacted or treatment goals have been met and the ecology of the family of origin has changed sufficiently to support the clinical advances. Reunification is also contingent upon the development and successful implementation of the safety plan. Generally, several successful visitations in which safety plans are adequately implemented should occur before youth and family members are permanently reunified. Often, the process of implementing safety plans in the natural ecology will lead to modifications that enhance the utility and effectiveness of the plan. Intensive MST home-based services continue through the reunification process and until the other overarching goals of treatment are achieved.

### Use of TFC in the Service of MST Treatment Goals

While safety is an overriding goal of treatment and is sometimes the reason youth are placed in foster care, TFC is more often used within the

MST continuum as a way to prevent more restrictive or longer term out-of-home placements. In such cases, TFC is used when less restrictive alternatives (e.g., team monitoring in the home) or kinship placements (e.g., with grandparents, with an older sister) are unavailable or clinically inappropriate. As with any clinical service provided within the MST continuum, TFC should always be implemented in the service of treatment goals pertaining to engagement, assessment, interventions, or overcoming barriers to treatment.

## TO FACILITATE ENGAGEMENT AND PREVENT PLACEMENT

Although TFC would not be used to facilitate engagement alone, this intervention might be used when lack of engagement places a youth at high risk of more intensive placement. For example, TFC was used for engagement purposes with a new MST family in which the single mother was not yet aligned with the therapist. The teenage daughter was at risk of placement in a juvenile justice facility if she tested positive for drugs on her weekly urine drug screens or violated curfew. As the therapist attempted to set mechanisms in place for the mother to increase her supervision of the youth, he recognized that maternal supervision was going to be severely lacking over the weekend due to multiple factors (e.g., low engagement, work schedule, three young children in the home, symptoms of dysthymia). Because the weekend presented a time of high risk for the daughter (e.g., she would have access to frequent drug parties in the neighborhood) and the mother refused less restrictive interventions (e.g., contacting extended family to help, the presence of a crisis caseworker to help supervise the youth during waking hours), the team and mother decided to place the youth in TFC for the weekend. This placement enabled the daughter to remain drug-free (and to pass her drug screen) and provided respite for the mother to facilitate engagement. Care was taken, however, to let the mother know that this respite was provided on a one-time-only basis and that in the future solutions that used indigenous or team resources would be prioritized.

## TO FACILITATE ASSESSMENT AND PREVENT PLACEMENT

TFC would not be used solely to facilitate assessment of a youth or family member, but might be used when the lack of a valid assessment places the youth at significant risk of out-of-home placement. For example, a father and his 15-year-old son had an extremely volatile and aggressive relationship that threatened the stability of the boy's placement. Unfortunately, the assessment of the determinants of the intense father–son hostility was impeded by the chaos and high levels of sibling conflict evident in the household. Because the family had just recently moved to town, indigenous respite could not be accessed to provide a cooling-down period that would facilitate an accurate assessment. A brief foster care placement with a family in the neighborhood was arranged to provide the MST team an opportunity to obtain assessment information concerning (1) the youth's response to caregivers who have strong parenting skills and (2) the structure and affect in the home when the son was not present. In the more controlled atmosphere provided by a few days of TFC respite, the MST team could better assess the contribution of various individual and environmental factors to the father–son hostility. This information was subsequently used to craft interventions to sustain the son in his natural ecology.

## TFC AS AN INTERVENTION

TFC is most commonly accessed by MST therapists for continuum youth when the clinical team is trying to assist caregivers in extinguishing violent and oppositional behavior in youth who have a long history of having such behavior reinforced by their family and context. When caregivers of such youth do not have the emotional (e.g., severe depression, borderline personality) or physical (e.g., elderly grandmother with heart disease) capacity to adhere to stringent behavioral plans and tolerate the extinction outbursts of oppositional behavior that can be expected, temporary placement in TFC may be an appropriate intervention. Again, care is taken to ensure that caregivers who are indigenous to the youth's ecology (e.g., church members, relatives) cannot fulfill these roles before the youth is placed in TFC. In such instances, the TFC parents are supported in implementing a behavioral plan that is similar to the one the team plans to put into place in the youth's home. When the team and foster parents have managed to get the youth's behavior under control, the team then works to transfer these treatment gains back into the natural ecology. In some instances, TFC parents meet with the family of origin to assist in transferring hope, information, and skills. The use of TFC to implement stringent behavioral plans draws on less restrictive placements and enhances the generalizability of outcomes obtained while in foster care.

## TO ADDRESS BARRIERS TO EFFECTIVE TREATMENT

At times, despite their best efforts, MST therapists are unable to move families toward clinically significant changes in behavior. Often, the barriers to treatment progress are highly embedded in the family's context (e.g., poverty, low social support) or may involve severe caregiver psychopathology (e.g., substance abuse, major depression). In some instances, when more indigenous caregiver resources are not available, TFC can be used to obtain the time needed to address serious limitations in caregiver capacity to parent effectively. For example, neighborhood-based TFC was used as a safe placement for a substance-abusing daughter while her cocaine-addicted mother attended a 6-week residential drug treatment program. While the mother was receiving drug rehabilitation, the MST team helped the foster parents maintain the teenager in her regular school and began implementing interventions for her own substance abuse problems. Upon the mother's return, she was reunited with her daughter and the team took responsibility for designing and implementing treatment services for the daughter and aftercare services for the mother.

## Case Example

Tom was a 14-year-old white male with both oppositional and internalizing symptoms. He had been physically and emotionally abused by his father and was subsequently placed in the home of his mother and stepfather by social services at the age of 13 years. In his mother's home, Tom had demonstrated increasingly aggressive behaviors, kicking holes in the walls and screaming loudly whenever limits were set. As a result of this behavior, Tom had been hospitalized on the psychiatric unit on five separate occasions and was at risk of long-term placement in a residential treatment facility when his family began MST.

Initially, team therapists and crisis caseworkers stayed with the family and youth around the clock during nonsleeping hours to assess Tom's acting-out behavior and assist the family in implementing safety and behavioral plans. Within a week, it became apparent that Tom would respond to a behavioral plan that could be followed by caregivers with a moderate level of skills. The team was successful in teaching these skills to the stepfather, and team members observed him implementing the skills successfully on several occasions. On the other hand, Tom's mother had great difficulty acquiring these skills and continued to have interactions with Tom that increased, rather than diminished, his aggressive behavior.

In working with the mother to better understand the fit of her poor implementation, the therapist and psychiatrist performed an individual evaluation. They concluded that she was suffering from PTSD and depression. These problems were directly impairing her ability to parent Tom effectively. For example, when Tom began to yell at his mother (the first sequence of behaviors that occurred when she tried to set limits), she experienced strong feelings of fear and anger (PTSD symptoms from

domestic violence by Tom's father). Without thinking, she would become unreasonably irritable and verbally aggressive. This, in turn, triggered Tom's escalation into a series of more violent verbal and physical
behaviors.

The therapist and psychiatrist used cognitive-behavioral therapy
and antidepressant medication to reduce the mother's symptoms. But it
became increasingly clear to them that she was too overwhelmed, depressed, and anxious to respond to treatment while in the process of trying to parent and supervise her son. Although the team provided extensive support to the stepfather and enlisted assistance from indigenous
resources (i.e., an aunt) to monitor Tom, his very aggressive behavior
continued to be exacerbated by problematic interactions with his mother.
Due to the overwhelming clinical demands that were being placed on the
MST team (i.e., 6–8 hours of in-home support each day), the added
stress on the family, and concern that the family would get evicted from
their apartment if the outbursts continued, a decision was made to place
Tom in TFC for 3–4 weeks.

The placement allowed the mother to have respite from the stimuli
triggering PTSD and depressive symptoms, and gave the CBT and psychopharmacological treatments time to take effect. The behavioral plan
for Tom was implemented in the TFC home. Care was taken to ensure
cross-family consistency in behavior. Importantly, Tom visited his family
of origin weekly and continued to attend the same school despite the 40-
minute drive this imposed on the families and team members. After approximately 5 weeks in the TFC home and several successful extended
visitations to resolve any difficulties in the safety plan, Tom was successfully reunited with his family and MST home-based treatment was continued.

## RESIDENTIAL AND PSYCHIATRIC
## INPATIENT PLACEMENTS

Consistent with the System of Care (SOC) Principles, an underlying philosophy of MST is that children should receive services within the least
restrictive and most normative environment that is clinically appropriate
(Principle 3; Stroul, 1988). While this belief is embedded in the zeitgeist
of the National Child and Adolescent Service System Program (CASSP)
SOC movement (Stroul & Friedman, 1986), the relevance of the least restrictive environment philosophy to MST also lies in the child mental
health services empirical literature. The evidence base supports the use
of ecological, community, and family-based services as preferred alternatives to treatment in restrictive settings for youth with serious emotional

and behavioral problems (Henggeler, Rowland, et al., 1999; Rivera & Kutash, 1994; U.S. Public Health Service, 2000). Importantly, this literature indicates that treatment in residential and inpatient settings, while secure, has little demonstrated effectiveness. Moreover, some data suggest that institution-based services may have detrimental effects on youth and their families (Burns, 1991; Elliott, 1998; U.S. Public Health Service, 2000). Yet, at times, use of highly restrictive placements is needed to treat significant individual symptoms in the youth (e.g., psychosis, mania) or to maintain the safety of youth or family members. Thus, MST continuum treatment teams need access to a range of clinical placements that span several levels of restrictiveness, including residential and psychiatric inpatient.

The purpose of residential or hospital placements within an MST continuum is to provide safe sites to treat youth when less restrictive options are not viable. In developing clinical protocols for the provision of services while youth are in such placements, three shifts from traditional institution-based practices have occurred. First and most important, *the MST treatment team maintains clinical responsibility for the youth* while he or she is in placement. Hence, the MST therapist, supervisor, and psychiatrist continue to provide direct treatment across all community and placement sites in the continuum. Such continuity in clinical decision making allows the team's ongoing assessment, intervention, and evaluation processes to continue uninterrupted and is critical in maintaining the focus on clinical outcomes. In addition, the clinical continuity helps the family to remain engaged with the treatment team, rather than having to negotiate relationships with multiple, and at times conflicting, providers. The second clinical shift is that *treatment for MST youth in these settings is systemic and geared toward enhancing the youth's functioning in the natural ecology.* This perspective differs from the traditional focus on individual pathology that characterizes most inpatient and residential facilities. Hence, individualized treatment plans are designed to be carried out for MST youths while in restrictive placements. These plans place a premium on developing behaviors that will be adaptive in the youth's natural ecology and often minimize the youth's interface with peers in the residential or inpatient setting. Likewise, and third, *MST youth are generally excluded from unit group activities.* Although this change is difficult to implement and sustain in residential and inpatient settings, a growing body of clinical research (Dishion et al., 1999) and clinical experience suggests that adolescents with serious behavior problems are particularly vulnerable to negative peer influences and that treatments that place groups of adolescents with behavioral problems together may do more harm than good (Arnold & Hughes, 1999; Poulin, Dishion, & Haas, 1999).

## When and Where to Place

Restrictive placements (e.g., in a hospital or residential treatment center) should only occur when the treatment team has determined that the clinical problem targeted for intervention (e.g., mania, psychosis, violence) is largely driven by individual factors that are appropriately treated in such settings (e.g., via medications, behavioral protocols). To the extent that the youth's problematic behavior is driven by contextual factors such as marital discord or poor parental monitoring, interventions should target the contexts and allow for the youth to be treated in more community-based settings (e.g., at home with clinical team observation, at the home of a relative, or with TFC). Thus, youth who are admitted into the inpatient psychiatric unit should present significant safety or treatment concerns that cannot be dealt with effectively by the family and clinical team in the community.

Moreover, as with respite, TFC, or other clinical services, the MST supervisor must ensure that the placement is occurring in the service of a treatment goal and that this goal cannot be achieved in a less restrictive setting (e.g., TFC, home of a relative). With this criterion met, the team attempts to place the youth in the least restrictive setting that can effectively address the reasons for placement. In deciding which placement is least restrictive, yet clinically appropriate, the supervisor considers site location (e.g., proximity to family, neighborhood), ability to facilitate youth interface with community, clinical needs of the youth, and staffing and patient characteristics of the placement setting. Often, more functional concerns (e.g., funding, bed availability) drive the decision.

## Roles of Team Members

The team psychiatrist is the clinical lead when youth are placed in residential or inpatient settings. The psychiatrist is the admitting physician on the psychiatric unit, provides the intake assessment, writes the treatment orders, and orchestrates treatment and discharge planning and implementation. Team members (e.g., therapist, crisis caseworker, family resource specialist) meet daily to specify intervention plans, write notes on the chart, and interface with unit treatment staff to ensure implementation of plans. Whenever possible, however, treatment team members provide services directly. Hence, the MST therapists as well as the supervisor and psychiatrist must obtain clinical privileges to provide services in the residential or inpatient settings that are part of the continuum.

The therapist's primary role while youth are in placement is to understand and attempt to resolve the factors that resulted in placement. Thus, the therapist assesses the individual, family, and systems factors driving the behaviors that resulted in placement and works with the supervisor and psychiatrist to develop appropriate interventions. Therapists often work harder when youth are in placement settings than when youth are at home because intensive interventions are being delivered across these settings. For example, therapists treat the youth in the facility, provide family therapy or other services to the family at home, and assist in communicating behavioral plans and providing clinical materials to residential staff who have contact with the youth.

## Case Example

This example highlights how an inpatient setting can be used in the service of MST treatment goals. Shequella was a 13-year-old African American female who was referred to the MST treatment team due to conduct disorder, marijuana abuse, depression, and running away. She had been suspended from school for threatening a teacher and was running away to the homes of older peers for a week or two at the time. An assessment of the fit of her behavior revealed poor parental monitoring and weak parent–child affective bonds as primary drivers. Thus, initial interventions targeted these problems by shoring up the mother's resources for monitoring (e.g., with support from crisis caseworkers and grandparents), helping the mother develop better parenting skills, and increasing positive affective experiences between mother and daughter.

As the mother became more adept at implementing the behavioral plans and accessing supports, the clinical team was able to diminish their involvement. Likewise, as Shequella's symptoms improved, she was allowed to earn developmentally appropriate increases in privileges. In planning for the possible reemergence of problems, however, the MST team developed a behavioral plan that outlined the consequences that would occur if Shequella ran away, used drugs (drug use was being monitored with weekly urine screens), or skipped school (daily report cards were being obtained from teachers).

Despite much improved behavior for 5 weeks, Shequella did not return home from school one day and remained missing for 2 weeks. After an extensive search involving police, family, and family friends, Shequella was located in the home of an 18-year-old "friend" who lived with roommates in an apartment frequented by substance-using young adults who engaged in criminal activities. Because Shequella was too angry and distraught to contract for safety, the MST team psychiatrist evaluated Shequella and decided to admit her to the inpatient psychiatric unit for further assessment of depression and running-away behavior that posed a risk of self harm. This decision was supported by the mother and the therapist, who were afraid that Shequella would run away again even if she was closely supervised.

Shequella was on the inpatient unit for 4 days. During this time, several interventions took place. Individually, she was assessed for depression and restarted on an antidepressant. To promote her work toward developing a safety plan that could be implemented at home, Shequella was placed on a room program in which she was required to complete a list of peers with whom she had contact while on runaway and to give their locations and phone numbers. The therapist determined the sequences of events that led to Shequella running away and what factors maintained this status. Shequella also received an adolescent medicine evaluation to rule out pregnancy or sexually transmitted disease. Because Shequella was easily influenced by deviant peers, she remained on the unit under close staff supervision and did not attend group therapies or activities. Rather, she completed assignments that directly impacted the reasons she had been placed on the unit (e.g., by listing triggers for running, writing apology letters to teachers, completing school work, setting individual goals for school) as part of her room program.

During family sessions, the therapist reviewed the sequence of events that lead to and sustained the running-away behavior with the mother and daughter. Together, the mother, therapist and Shequella established a new safety plan. As part of this plan, the mother and therapist called and visited the list of peers provided by Shequella. The mother took out a restraining order on the young men who were 18 years or older and informed them of her intention to have them arrested if they were seen with Shequella again. After several days of hard work, a safety plan was in place that allowed the mother to safely maintain Shequella in her home. Thus, the inpatient stay provided an opportunity to safely negotiate changes in the youth (e.g., medication) and social ecology (e.g., list of hideouts, support from law enforcement) that would increase the probability that Shequella would maintain appropriate behavior upon discharge.

## PSYCHOPHARMACOLOGICAL INTERVENTIONS

One of the primary modifications made to enhance the effectiveness of MST for youth at risk of out-of-home placement due to mental health problems has been the integration of psychiatrists into the clinical team. Psychiatrists play an essential role in helping to ensure that youth and their family members receive appropriate psychiatric and, if indicated, medical care. Specifically, team psychiatrists provide psychiatric evaluations of youth and family members; clinical consultation with the MST treatment team; community liaison with outside physicians concerning medical or psychiatric care of youth, caregivers, and family members; and emergency psychiatric evaluations (e.g., in the emergency room, in a shelter). In addition, the team's primary psychiatrist is responsible for assisting with the development of protocols to manage aggressive behavior in the community and procedures for dealing with safety concerns. Often, the psychiatrist is responsible for signing certain of the therapist's clinical notes and ensuring adequate charting of crisis assessments and interventions.

One of the most important roles psychiatrists play is the implementation of psychopharmacological interventions for youth and, when indicated, family members. As with all clinical interventions implemented within the MST framework, care is taken to ensure that psychopharmacological interventions are guided by research findings. Thus, MST psychiatrists are expected to have a working knowledge of the empirical data supporting the use of pharmacological interventions for psychiatric disorders in children and adults. While the literature for children is somewhat limited, many studies support the use of stimulants in youth with ADHD (Burns, Compton, Egger, & Farmer, 2000; Greenhill et al., 1996), and some data support the nontricyclic antidepressants for treating childhood depression and anxiety (Emslie, Walkup, Pliszka, & Ernst, 1999; Weisz & Jensen, 1999). Hence, when helping therapists intervene with these problems, physicians are expected to diagnose appropriately, know which medication choices and dosing patterns represent empirically established bases, and monitor concurrent medical and psychiatric conditions as indicated.

In light of the significant gaps in the empirical literature concerning appropriate medications for many of the childhood conditions (Weisz & Jensen, 1999), psychiatrists are also expected to maintain a basic understanding of the prevailing consensus of "best practice" procedures and to follow these as closely as possible for those conditions in which more empirically driven data are not available. Likewise, because team psychiatrists may need to provide evaluations for caregivers in more than 50% of the families receiving MST, a thorough understanding of the adult treatment literature is essential. To aid MST psychiatrists in developing protocols and maintaining an up-to-date understanding of the empirical literature, linkages with consulting MST child psychiatrists are maintained through the weekly telephone consultation that is part of the quality assurance protocol described in Chapter 2. As part of this process, the consulting MST psychiatrist provides materials and references that are salient to applying efficacious treatments (e.g., stimulants for ADHD) in real-world settings (Hughes et al., 1999; Pliszka, Carlson, & Swanson, 1999; Pliszka et al., 2000a) and assists with the development of practical protocols to address clinical dilemmas relating to medications or other issues that require psychiatric expertise (e.g., safety, risk reduction).

## CONCLUSION

During the course of treatment in traditional MST home-based programs, situations arise that might benefit from the planful and judicious
use of placements. Similarly, not all families are empowered to address
their own mental health needs by the conclusion of 3–5 months of intensive services. The use of an evidence-based continuum of care that maintains the continuity of clinical decision making and high levels of quality
assurance holds the potential to achieve "the Holy Grail" of children's
mental health services: improved clinical- and services-related outcomes
at reduced cost. Moreover, the integration of evidence-based psychopharmacological interventions with intensive ecological treatments
might provide an extremely useful synergy. As discussed in Chapter 8,
studies are in progress to evaluate these possibilities.

# CHAPTER 7

# Case Examples

Through the use of three detailed case examples, this chapter
depicts the complex and multifaceted nature of providing
broad-based treatment to youths with serious emotional disturbance. It also emphasizes the importance of developing indigenous supports and integrating these with evidence-based interventions. Moreover, this chapter provides a realistic appraisal
of the ongoing mental health needs of youths presenting the
most serious clinical problems.

This chapter provides a broad and relatively detailed depiction of
the implementation of MST with youths presenting serious mental
health difficulties and their families. Three case examples are presented
from a clinical trial adapting MST to treat youth experiencing acute psychiatric distress (Henggeler, Rowland, et al., 1999). Client names and
identifying information have been changed to protect confidentiality.

## JONATHAN

This case highlights the inherent complexity of treating youth who are
experiencing a psychiatric emergency in the community, and the range of

resources often required to achieve clinical improvement with such children and their families. In addition, this case provides a good example of the mobilization and extended use of indigenous supports needed to safely and effectively maintain a child presenting serious mental health and behavioral problems in the community (Principles 2 and 9).

## Presenting Information

Jonathan, a 14-year-old Caucasian male, was enrolled in MST as an alternative to psychiatric hospitalization after presenting in crisis to the emergency room. Jonathan was brought to the emergency room by the police as a result of physical aggression toward his mother (i.e., he chased her with a bat) and threats to harm himself (i.e., he threatened to run in front of a car). During the weeks leading up to the evaluation, Jonathan's mother had observed a dramatic increase in his behavioral problems. Jonathan had been more disruptive in school, and had threatened his teacher and peers as well as himself, stating that he wanted to jump from a second-story window in the school.

## Intake Assessment and History

Jonathan lived with his mother and 13-year-old brother, Cedric, in a low-income and high-crime housing development. During the assessment, family members were cooperative and appeared to get along well with each other. Jonathan had one previous referral to the emergency room several years ago, which resulted in 5 days of hospitalization and minimal follow-up at a local community mental health center. Jonathan had an extensive history of poor achievement, aggression, and classroom disruption at school that had become more pronounced in recent years. For example, Jonathan had been expelled from school several times for verbal and physical aggression toward peers, teachers, and school staff. Unfortunately, these expulsions precluded attendance in regular school settings and required Jonathan to attend an alternative school for students with behavior problems.

During the assessment, Jonathan acknowledged the reasons for his referral and endorsed symptoms of depression (e.g., mood lability, irritability), but denied suicidal ideation. Jonathan admitted that he sometimes threatened to hurt himself to "get attention," and reported that his primary difficulty was his mother, who "makes me mad and won't stop picking on me." Jonathan denied a history of physical or sexual abuse, drug or alcohol use, school problems, or maternal alcohol or drug use. Jonathan's brother, Cedric, reported doing well in school (i.e., good grades, no referrals for inappropriate behaviors), and indicated that he got along well with his peers and was a member of the school band.

According to the mother's report, the family had a history of substance abuse in both parents, domestic violence, and schizophrenia in a paternal uncle. Jonathan's father, who lived with the family sporadically, had a history of crack cocaine addiction and considerable involvement with the criminal justice system. The mother reported that Jonathan's father was physically abusive toward her and had received a 5-year prison term for selling drugs. This prison term had ended 5 months previously, and he was in the community on parole. Both boys had witnessed the domestic disputes and had been physically abused by the father in the past when they tried to intervene on their mother's behalf. Mother acknowledged an extensive history of alcohol dependence, but had received few mental health or substance abuse services. She reported sobriety for much of the past 5 years, but described a pronounced increase in "nerve problems," some difficulties "thinking straight," and "trouble staying off the bottle" since her husband's release from prison. Further exploration of her current psychiatric difficulties revealed disorganized thoughts, severe anxiety with hyperarousal consistent with PTSD, and mood lability and sleep disturbance consistent with depression.

In addition to the mother's psychiatric symptoms and concern for Jonathan's problems, several additional stressors were identified. These centered on financial problems as a result of the mother's recent unemployment. Due to limited financial resources, the family did not have a phone or reliable means of transportation, and their utilities were about to be discontinued. An additional stressor identified by the mother was social isolation. She felt ostracized by her extended family, including her mother and sister, whom she described as recently refusing to help her and her children.

## Strengths

Despite the aforementioned stressors and the significant psychiatric difficulties exhibited by Jonathan and his mother, several strengths (Principle 2) were evident that could be used to facilitate treatment outcome (see Figure 7.1). For example, Jonathan's personable demeanor and social skills had prompted several adults to take an active interest in his wellbeing. Despite his history of verbal and physical aggression, Jonathan had elicited only one formal criminal charge, suggesting protective factors operating in his life. The immediate family had a strong affective bond, and the mother was motivated to receive help to address her own mental health problems as well as her son's. Although relations with the

| STRENGTHS | NEEDS |
|---|---|

**Individual**

| | |
|---|---|
| • Insight into family conflicts. | • Depressed, periodically suicidal, mood lability, and irritability. |
| • History of using time-outs. | |
| • Seeks and responds well to adult attention. | • Physically aggressive toward mother, peers, school staff. |
| • Personable and easy to engage. | • Disruptive at school. |
| • Motivated to control aggression. | • Borderline intelligence. |
| • History of only one criminal charge. | • Pending criminal charge for shoplifting. |

**Family**

| | |
|---|---|
| • Mother motivated to obtain services for herself and children. | • Maternal substance abuse and psychopathology. |
| • Strong affective bond between mother and children. | • History of physical violence between family members. |
| • Mother has a history of using time-outs at neighbor and respite with sister. | • Father is a chronic criminal offender. |
| | • Minimal bond with younger brother. |
| • Younger brother does well in school. | • Poor family boundaries. |
| • Extended family available in the community. | • Mother has limited parenting skills. |

**Peers**

| | |
|---|---|
| • Some friends at school participate in prosocial activities. | • Most peers are unknown by the mother and extended family. |
| • Several neighborhood peers participate in prosocial activities at the community recreational center. | • Peers at school often tease J about his mother's behavior and the sexual orientation of his brother; this often leads to fights. |
| | • Criminal charge occurred when J shoplifted with peers. |

**School**

| | |
|---|---|
| • J enjoys going to school and attends school regularly. | • This is the third year in a row J has been considered for expulsion during the first term. |
| • J has a positive bond with his guidance counselor. | • J is physically aggressive with peers and select school staff. |
| • This counselor is invested in J and sought assistance from mental health providers. | • J failed second and third grades. |
| • Principal withdrew expulsion plans and is willing to work with MST team. | • The school has used ineffective and reinforcing behavioral plans to decrease J's aberrant behavior. |
| | • There is a long-standing adversarial relationship between the mother and the school. |

**Community**

| | |
|---|---|
| • Recreation center located near the home. | • Low-income, high-crime neighborhood. |
| | • Drug activity rampant. |
| • There is an adult at the recreation center with a vested interest in J (Mr. Jones). | • Neighbors with schizophrenia enter and leave the family's home without permission. |
| • Local church picks up youth at least once a week for afterschool prosocial activities. | • Area drug dealers have tried to recruit J into the drug trade. |

**FIGURE 7.1.** Systemic strengths and needs: Jonathan.

nearby extended family were strained, they had previously provided respite and frequently encouraged Jonathan's mother to obtain help for her substance use problems.

## Safety

In light of Jonathan's acute homicidal and suicidal threats, the initial goal of treatment was to ensure his safety and the safety of members of his immediate family, classmates, and school personnel. Toward this end, the MST treatment team, comprised of master's-level therapists, bachelor's-level crisis caseworkers, a clinical child psychologist, and a child psychiatrist, reviewed the intake assessment information provided by the therapist and psychiatrist to identify factors that were contributing to Jonathan's risk of harm to himself and others (Principle 1). Due to the substantial risk of homicide and suicide posed by the presence of firearms in the home, the initial safety plan for all MST youth requires home checks for weapons. Hence, the home was checked for bats, sharp objects that could be used as weapons (e.g., knives), and guns. In addition, a check was conducted for the presence of potentially dangerous medications. The mother was assisted in removing all potentially harmful items from the home.

MST safety plans should provide very specific details of who will participate and what each participant will do to maintain the child's safety. In the present case, the team felt that Jonathan could be maintained safely in the community with appropriate support. In such instances, the treatment team is responsible for identifying who may be able to participate in the safety plan and determining if the individuals have the skills and resources needed to be effective. Hence, the therapist and crisis caseworker interviewed key individuals in Jonathan's social ecology (Principles 2, 3, and 9) to assess their potential to help the clinical team. Mr. Jones, a resident advisor with the local housing authority and the director of the local recreation center, and Mr. Tyme, a neighbor, agreed to monitor Jonathan and be available for respite. A maternal aunt, Sheila, was also contacted and agreed to participate in the safety plan (Principle 9).

The safety plan included several components that integrated informal and formal supports. During the first week of treatment, 24-hour-a-day adult supervision and monitoring were provided by members of the clinical team and adults in Jonathan's ecology. Building on Jonathan's facility in seeking and responding favorably to attention from Mr. Jones, Mr. Tyme, and Aunt Sheila, these individuals were used to provide monitoring and brief periods of respite if Jonathon became verbally aggressive, as this often preceded physical aggression. Second, a schedule was developed for the community supports (i.e., Mr. Jones, Mr. Tyme, Aunt Sheila) and MST team members to periodically check Jonathan's home throughout the day to monitor his behavior and support his mother. Third, Jonathon's mother agreed that if he became agitated, that she would allow him to access this support system and "take a time-out." Finally, if Jonathan could not calm down within 30 minutes of the time-out, the mother or other members of the community support team would contact the therapist on call. The MST therapist would arrive on-site, assess the situation, and arrange appropriate interventions. These included the capacity to transport Jonathan to the local emergency room for evaluation by the MST psychiatrist if indicated (Principles 3 and 4).

### Fit Assessment

During the initial assessment, no obvious proximal factors seemed immediately relevant to Jonathan's aggressive behavior and suicidal threats. Based on information obtained for the Initial Assessment Form, however, the treatment team hypothesized that several more distal factors were either directly or indirectly influencing Jonathan's difficulties

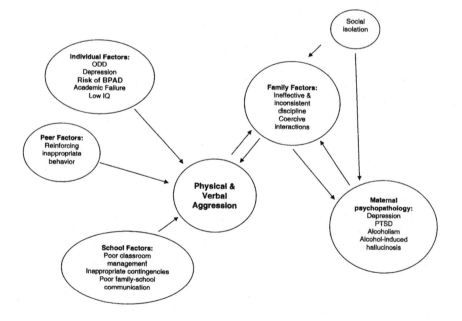

**FIGURE 7.2.** Jonathan's fit assessment.

(see Figure 7.2). Hypothesized fit factors (Principle 1) included (1) modeling aggression (e.g., witnessing domestic violence, physical abuse); (2) school failure (e.g., borderline intelligence, inappropriate classroom placement, achievement deficits, poor classroom management by his teachers); (3) association with deviant peers (e.g., shoplifting with a group of peers, recruitment by area drug dealers, alternative school placement); (4) weak behavioral contingencies at home and at school; (5) individual psychopathology (e.g., oppositional defiant disorder, depression [Children's Depression Inventory score in the moderate range]); (6) parental neglect/abuse (e.g., maternal psychopathology, paternal criminal and abusive behavior); and (7) family conflict (e.g., parent–child difficulties, marital problems). Developing a well-specified MST treatment plan (Principles 4, 5, and 8) required a comprehensive assessment of both proximal and distal factors associated with Jonathan's referral behaviors—garnered through direct observation of Jonathan at home and at school as well as from the reports of key members of his social ecology (e.g., family, teachers, informal supports).

## FAMILY

Because the proximal antecedents to Jonathan's aggressive and suicidal behavior were not clearly understood during the initial assessment, a more comprehensive assessment strategy was integrated into the initial 24-hour/7-day safety plan (Principle 5) developed for the first week. This strategy allowed direct observation of Jonathan in his natural environment as well as an adult presence to respond immediately to homicidal or suicidal threats. A tracking form was developed for those observing Jonathan to document any instance of verbal or physical aggression, suicidal threats, immediate (e.g., social/interpersonal interactions, mood states) or distal (e.g., argument with his mother the night before) antecedents to problem behavior, and the consequences given to the problem behavior (e.g., attention, escape/avoidance). In addition, the therapist completed a mental status exam and assessed Jonathan's suicidal ideation and his mother's alcohol use and anxiety symptoms. This integration of assessment into the safety plan enabled the treatment team to identify contextual or individual factors contributing directly and indirectly to Jonathan's homicidal and suicidal behavior (Principles 4 and 5).

After observing Jonathan and his family during the first week of treatment and reviewing the daily tracking form completed by multiple informants, the MST team discovered a distinct pattern to his aggressive behavior at home. Verbal and physical aggression were correlated with coercive interactions between Jonathan and his mother. For example, during one safety check-in, Mr. Jones observed Jonathan's mother frantically calling for him and his brother. Although the boys were playing appropriately with other children in the neighborhood, the mother, for no apparent reason, began to plead with them to return home. When Jonathan and his brother ignored her, she responded by repeating the request more vehemently. She then started crying and trying to persuade them to return home. When these efforts failed, she became more agitated and physical, grabbing and pulling her sons by their arms. After dragging Jonathan and Cedric home, she made them sit in the living room with her and not move. Following a brief period of compliance, the boys "slipped out" without any comment from the mother. This pattern of "command–compliance interaction" between Jonathan and his mother is common between parents and defiant children (Barkley, 1997), and was the most consistent pattern deduced from the daily tracking form and anecdotal evidence from members of the safety team. What remained unclear, however, was the antecedents that prompted the mother's frantic searching behavior, followed by apparent indifference to the boys' presence or absence.

To further to assess the fit of the mother's behavior, the therapist used two assessment strategies: (1) interviewing the mother and significant others (e.g., her sisters), and (2) observing the mother at high-risk times for coercive interactions to detect overt and covert antecedents to her behavior. Independent interviews with the mother and her sisters revealed that the mother frequently became very anxious and fearful for the children's welfare. The mother and her sisters hypothesized that her reactions were due to distress (i.e., PTSD) associated with chronic domestic violence. Furthermore, the aunts reported that the mother frequently "starts stuff with the kids when she is in these moods." The women confirmed the mother's use of alcohol, but denied any concerns about alcohol abuse or dependence. On three occasions that the therapist observed coercive interactions, however, she smelled alcohol on the mother. In contrast, the therapist did not detect alcohol use on occasions when there were no coercive interactions. Hence, the assessments supported the view that Jonathan's behavior problems were precipitated by coercive interactions between him and his mother secondary to her drinking and anxiety.

## SCHOOL

Although the aforementioned assessment provided a solid start to understanding Jonathan's aggressive and suicide-threatening behavior at home, such behavior at school remained unexplained. Here, classroom observations and interviews with his teacher and her aide suggested that Jonathan's aberrant school behavior was being maintained by several sources of reinforcement (Principles 1 and 8). When the teacher asked Jonathan to complete school work, he became increasingly oppositional and threatening, particularly when given math assignments or asked to read aloud in class. In response, the teacher would sometimes allow Jonathan to leave the classroom, thereby negatively reinforcing (i.e., removing a negative stimulus, school work) his oppositional behavior. If the teacher demanded that Jonathan complete the assigned work, then his behavior would escalate to threats to kill himself. These threats would then prompt his teacher to remove him from class. Thus, in both scenarios, Jonathan's oppositional behavior was being reinforced by allowing him to escape from or avoid unpleasant school tasks. Moreover, it is important to note that the teacher's behavior toward Jonathan was also being maintained by negative reinforcement: when Jonathan disrupted the classroom, she would remove him, and the disruption would cease.

Jonathan's oppositional behavior also seemed to be maintained by two sources of positive reinforcement: adult and peer attention. When Jonathan became agitated or oppositional his teacher would sometimes allow him "time-outs" with Mr. Perry, a very personable staff member whom he liked. Consequently, one function of Jonathan's oppositional behavior was to allow him to spend time with a favored school staff member. Consistent with the deviancy training hypothesis (Dishion et al., 1999), another function of Jonathan's aberrant classroom behavior was the positive reactions elicited by his alternative-school classmates. In addition, two setting events were associated with days that Jonathan was more likely to behave oppositionally: coercive interactions with his mother the previous evening and poor reading and math skills. Thus, Jonathan's aberrant school behavior was associated with proximal positive (i.e., adult and peer attention) and negative (i.e., escape from aversive school tasks) reinforcement as well as with more distal setting events (i.e., coercive interactions with his mother).

## SUMMARY AND OVERARCHING GOALS

The fit analyses identified several factors directly and indirectly related to Jonathan's difficulties at home and at school (see Figure 7.2). The therapist formed the following hypothesis: Jonathan is most likely to become aggressive at school when (1) his teacher asks him to do math assignments or read aloud in class, and (2) peers laugh at his behavior or he has access to Mr. Perry following misbehavior. In addition, (3) Jonathan's behavioral difficulties seem to be primed or exacerbated by coercive interactions at home, which are associated with maternal psychopathology and substance use. The resulting treatment plan, therefore, focused on these controlling influences to address a relatively consistent set of treatment goals. The mother wanted Jonathan to stop being physically and verbally aggressive toward her. Jonathan wanted his family to stop fighting and to go to school. And the teacher wanted to eliminate Jonathan's disruptive behavior and suicidal threats at school.

## Family and Individual Interventions

### ENGAGEMENT

To address these overarching goals, the therapist first had to engage the mother in treatment. Because the mother was highly concerned about the possibility of the Department of Social Services (DSS) removing the children from the home, this issue was addressed first. With the mother's consent, the therapist contacted DSS and learned of their ongoing involvement with the family and concerns regarding maternal mental health and substance abuse problems as well as the family's social isolation. With this information in hand, the therapist was able to help the mother to understand that therapeutic progress in these areas was probably the best way to ensure that her children would not be removed from the home by DSS (Principles 2 and 9).

### FOCUSING ON THE MOTHER AND BUILDING
### INDIGENOUS SUPPORTS

Following this engagement strategy (i.e., working with the mother to make the changes needed to keep her children in the home) a treatment plan targeting maternal substance abuse and anxiety (Principle 4) was developed. The initial components included a psychiatric evaluation and substance abuse treatment using aspects of Budney and Higgins's evidence-based community reinforcement approach (CRA; Budney & Higgins, 1998). Because the mother was apprehensive about an office evaluation, the therapist arranged for the team psychiatrist to meet with her at home. At the time of the assessment, the mother was severely impaired due to alcohol consumption and a mixture of psychotic, anxiety, and PTSD symptoms. The diagnostic impression of the physician was psychosis induced either by alcohol intoxication or withdrawal as well as PTSD and depression. Although the psychiatrist felt that the mother needed psychiatric hospitalization due to the severity and chronicity of her mental health and substance abuse problems, she refused hospitalization. She did agree, however, to work with the therapist to attempt to cut back on her alcohol use. The first and most important aspect of this treatment was her agreement to allow frequent checks of her vital signs to rule out alcohol withdrawal, and to consent to go to the emergency room with the therapist if these checks revealed unstable or worsening symptoms of withdrawal. The mother also agreed to let her sister, Sheila, monitor her sons over the weekend until she was more physically stable. Toward this end, components of CRA were incorporated into the mother's treatment plan, including a functional analysis of her drinking behavior (Principle 1), a self-management plan targeting fit factors identified in the functional analysis, and alcohol refusal skills.

A functional analysis of the mother's drinking behavior revealed that important triggers were feelings of anxiety associated with thoughts about her experiences with domestic violence and worries about her children's safety, which were especially acute when she was alone. To address her anxiety symptoms, the therapist began relaxation training and systematic desensitization, developed a safety plan that included daily check-ins with the therapist (the mother felt this would be helpful), and began rallying an indigenous support network to decrease the amount of time the mother spent alone. As part of the CRA approach, significant others were asked to reinforce the mother's efforts at abstinence. After receiving a release of information, the therapist contacted other members of the extended family to garner support for the mother's efforts at abstinence. Thus, family treatment focused on (1) pulling in the maternal grandmother and aunts to provide more day-to-day help in monitoring the children and ensuring that their basic needs were met, and (2) involving the maternal grandmother and aunts in the mother's substance treatment (Principles 7 and 9).

Unfortunately, after approximately 4 weeks of treatment, the mother continued coercive interactions with Jonathan and his brother that escalated and bordered on physical abuse, and her drinking increased to almost daily intoxication. As the mother's drinking increased, she became severely impaired and continued to refuse inpatient treatment. Although the therapist continued to try to address the mother's drinking on an outpatient basis, a report had to be made to DSS concerning the mother's physical aggression toward Jonathan. If Jonathan and his brother were to safely remain in the community, other family members would need to assume responsibility for their care (Principles 2 and 9).

## SHIFTING CARE TO THE EXTENDED FAMILY

The therapist then focused on helping the mother through the child abuse reporting process and consulting with the extended family to take temporary custody of the children. The mother was encouraged to contact DSS (with the therapist) and arrange a family meeting with her mother and sisters. The therapist educated the mother about the DSS reporting process and role-played the process with her. At the family meeting, the family decided that the boys would live with their grandmother temporarily, which would keep DSS from placing them out of the family. The aunts, while supportive of their mother's decision to take temporary custody, were initially adamant about not having further involvement with their sister. The aunts did not want to "enable" their sister's substance abuse and were concerned that their mother receive much-needed financial support. To address the aunts' concerns, the therapist arranged funding to help the grandmother meet the boys' basic needs via a combination of DSS contributions and local church donations, and then educated the aunts about the use of the probate court if they were concerned about their sister's safety and that of her children (Principles 5 and 8). The therapist sought and received agreement from the aunts to continue to participate in their sister's substance abuse treatment. Finally, the family developed, with the therapist's support, a detailed plan listing criteria for Jonathan and his brother to return home (e.g., the mother must be abstinent for 30 days).

The DSS referral, concomitant with encouragement from her mother and therapist and her sisters' threat of having her "committed," seemed to hasten the mother's acceptance of an inpatient substance abuse evaluation. After completing a 5-day inpatient detoxification program, the mother was diagnosed with alcohol-induced psychosis and PTSD, and agreed to complete a day treatment program. Unfortunately, the mother failed to attend the aftercare program and returned to heavy drinking soon after being discharged from the hospital.

Once Jonathan started living with his grandmother, the therapist assessed her parenting strengths and needs, and developed a treatment plan informed by this assessment (Principle 1). The basics of this plan were consistent with the conceptual analyses discussed previously.

## Individual Interventions for Jonathan

Jonathan had a history of one past psychiatric hospitalization for symptoms of depression and ODD several years prior. He reported minimal response to antidepressant treatment. His follow-up care with the local community mental health center was sporadic. At intake into MST, Jonathan's symptoms were consistent with major depressive disorder in that he was experiencing a disturbance in sleep, mood, energy, and appetite; and his score on the Children's Depression Inventory (Kovacs, 1992) was moderately elevated. While demonstrating some anxiety symptoms, he did not meet full criteria for PTSD or any other anxiety disorder. His history did not support the diagnosis of ADHD or thought disorder. Jonathan denied suicidal intent or plan and had a history of threatening suicidal acts but had no past attempts. He easily contracted for safety and aligned quickly with the therapist and team in implementing his own safety plan.

The MST psychiatrist initially started Jonathan on a low dose of a selective serotonin reuptake inhibitor (SSRI) antidepressant, as these have the most data to support their use in adolescents (Hughes et al., 1999). The therapist and the psychiatrist developed a quick list of symptoms to have Jonathan rate on a daily basis. The therapist administered the Children's Depression Inventory every other week. These data points along with Jonathan's subjective reports to the therapist were used to adjust his medication dose over the first 8 weeks. Despite increasing the medication to an adequate dose, Jonathan's individual symptoms did not improve; rather, he became more irritable, dysphoric, and agitated. As these symptoms coincided with his mother's hospitalization, the team initially attributed the problems to psychosocial factors. Yet Jonathan's individual symptoms continued to deteriorate despite improvement in his psychosocial situation (i.e., living with grandmother). Another psychiatric evaluation at this point revealed symptoms more consistent with mania in that Jonathan was irritable, more disorganized, and somewhat grandiose. Although he did not meet full criteria for bipolar affective disorder, given his family history of thought disorder and severe substance abuse disorders, as well as his increased mood lability on the SSRI, a decision was made to discontinue the antidepressant and place Jonathan on a mood stabilizer. Although lithium has the most data to support its use as a mood stabilizer in adolescents with bipolar affective disorder, the treatment team was concerned that the family would not be able to safely adhere to the dosing and blood-level monitoring regimen required to safely take lithium. Thus, Jonathan was started on valproic acid.

Continued careful monitoring of both depressive and manic symptoms over the next 6 weeks resulted in an adequate serum level, which corresponded with improved mood and affect. Importantly, Jonathan's teachers noticed a marked improvement in his symptoms of irritability and distractibility on this new medication. The optimization of Jonathan's medication regimen coincided with improvements in his living conditions and implementation of the classroom behavioral management plan discussed subsequently. Hence, the extent to which the medication contributed to improvement was difficult to fully assess. The MST psychiatrist, nevertheless, continued to see Jonathan periodically to assess serum levels of the medication and to monitor symptom improvement.

## School Interventions

Prior to Jonathan's removal from his mother's home, his behavioral problems at school had escalated and he was recommended for expulsion. Although Jonathan had a 504 plan in place, theoretically protecting him from expulsion by federal law, his behavior was so disruptive that the school feared for his safety. To address the school's concerns, an MST intervention plan was developed, with recommendations from Jonathan's teacher and a school administrator, that provided emergency consultation from the therapist and an immediate family response to any school crisis, as well as contingency management (Principle 6). Following recommendations for implementing school-related interventions discussed in an earlier chapter, the therapist arranged a meeting between the teacher, assistant principle, and mother to (1) identify the school's concerns and solicit their help in developing a treatment plan; (2) allow the MST treatment team ample opportunity to develop and implement the interventions, thereby delaying the expulsion; and (3) develop a strategy to monitor daily school behavior.

When the school was satisfied (i.e., engaged) that the therapist and family members would be immediately available to take Jonathan home, if needed, the therapist focused on changing school contingencies identified in the fit assessment as functionally related to his behavioral problems at school. Following the development and implementation of a "Daily Report Card," contingencies were rearranged at school such that escape-motivated behavior was met with aversive consequences and compliance was rewarded. For example, Jonathan's oppositional and aggressive behavior no longer allowed him to escape aversive school tasks, but resulted in (1) response cost and positive practice (e.g., completing assigned tasks and an additional assignment, apologizing publicly for his inappropriate behavior), (2) disappointment expressed by Mr. Perry and his grandmother, and (3) aversive consequences at home (e.g., loss of privileges such as television, video games, or outside play; writing sentences). Compliance with class assignments and teacher directives, however, were rewarded with adult attention (e.g., time with Mr. Perry, praise from grandmother and aunts) and access to privileges at home. The MST therapist was responsible for tracking each component of the school plan to ensure appropriate implementation and to determine whether the plan was decreasing Jonathan's behavioral problems (Principle 8).

Peer reinforcement of Jonathan's disruptive behavior also needed to be addressed. Classroom observations suggested that reinforcement of inappropriate behavior by Jonathan's classmates was associated with two factors (Principle 1). The teacher had a limited range of classroom management skills in her repertoire, relying mostly on threats and coercion. In addition, she had minimal administrative or aide support to manage a challenging group of students, each with a history of acting out in classroom settings. To address these factors, several interventions were implemented. First, the therapist engaged the teacher in Jonathan's behavioral plan and solicited her input in modifying the plan as needed. Second, the therapist shared articles on classroom management with the teacher, after she requested this information. Finally, the therapist, with the assistance of her clinical supervisor, helped the teacher develop and implement group contingencies to augment her behavioral expectations via peer pressure. Using elements of the ADHD Classroom Kit (Anhalt, McNeil, & Bahl, 1998), an empirically supported method of managing disruptive classroom behavior, the therapist taught the teacher how to impose group contingencies. Essentially, the class was divided into four groups. Each group could earn "Happy Faces" for following rules and teacher instructions or "Sad Faces" for rule violations and noncompliance. Throughout the day, groups receiving more happy faces than sad faces earned tangible rewards (e.g., 5 minutes of playtime, treats, access to computer games).

## Outcomes

Jonathan and his brother are now living with their grandmother. Jonathan is exhibiting fewer behavior problems across contexts due to the more stable living environment provided by the grandmother and familial support for following the home and school behavioral plans. Unfortunately, however, Jonathan's mother continues to drink heavily and often calls Jonathan while intoxicated, which usually precipitates problems at school the next day. DSS found substantive evidence of abuse and neglect, and transferred custody to the grandmother. Despite strong clinical gains, Jonathan continues to exhibit sporadic episodes of disruptive behavior with no clear antecedents. These episodes tax the grandmother, but can be managed with the emotional and respite support provided by her daughters. At discharge, Jonathan's mental health care was transferred to a school-based treatment team staffed with therapists and a psychiatrist from the local mental health center.

## BRENT

The case of Brent provides good examples of the key role that parents can play in attenuating serious emotional and behavioral problems as well as the integration of evidence-based pharmacological treatment into MST psychosocial protocols.

## Presenting Information

Brent was an 11-year-old African American male who lived with his father, 15-year-old sister, and 6-year-old brother. A home-based counselor from the local community mental health center referred Brent for psychiatric hospitalization because of her concerns with his increasingly aggressive and oppositional behavior. During her most recent home visit, for example, Brent had become increasingly frustrated and verbally abusive toward his father as he made appropriate demands regarding his son's behavior. Brent became so enraged that he grabbed a hammer, started threatening to hit his younger brother on the head, and then barricaded himself in his room. After removing the bedroom door, the counselor had to restrain Brent as he attempted to physically strike the counselor and family members. When Brent was unable to calm down, he was transported to the emergency room of the psychiatric hospital for evaluation. Due to Brent's escalating violent behavior, his potential to harm family members, and his failure to respond to intensive community-based mental health interventions, the emergency room physician recommended acute inpatient psychiatric hospitalization. At that point, the family was seen by the MST team.

## Intake Assessment and History

During the intake assessment (see Figure 7.3), Brent's father identified three areas of concern: (1) Brent's aggressive behavior at home, (2) his own psychosocial functioning, and (3) problems with his other children. Regarding Brent, the father described a 2-year history of severe aggressive behavior marked by physical and verbal assaults directed toward his siblings, especially his older sister. The father reported that Brent had become increasingly oppositional at home, but only had problems with impulsivity at school. He was receiving medication for ADHD. The father acknowledged that their home and family life were chaotic and that little structure was provided for the children because he worked nights for a telemarketing service and was frequently out of the home. Due to the practicalities of being a socially isolated single parent, the father gave his 15-year-old daughter responsibility for much of the parenting duties such as preparing evening meals, monitoring Brent' homework and curfew compliance, and managing her youngest brother. As such, the older sister was placed in an inescapable path of conflict with Brent. Brent and his older sister argued often, and these arguments were escalating to physical violence. Violence directed toward his sister resulted in two previous psychiatric hospitalizations for Brent as well as referral to a psychiatric day treatment program.

During his most recent hospitalization, Brent was started on a medication regimen to treat anxiety and ADHD. Unfortunately, the medications were only mildly effective in controlling his behavior at home. Brent, however, showed context specificity in his aberrant behavior. At

| STRENGTHS | NEEDS |
|---|---|
| **Individual** | |
| • Personable, assertive, and goal-directed. | • Oppositional and frequently tests limits with father and sister. |
| • Responds well to structure/contingencies. | • Exhibits poor frustration tolerance and poor impulse control. |
| • Problem-solved safety plan and accurately identified his own problem behaviors. | • History of violence toward sister. |
| | • Only problem-solving strategy at home is the use of anger and aggression. |
| • Aggressive behavior limited to the home. | • Diagnosed with ADHD and ODD. |
| • No criminal history. | |
| **Family** | |
| • Father works and provides for his family's basic needs. | • Father works the night shift and is away from home during high-risk times. |
| • Father is invested in helping his children. | • Father is frequently tired, possibly depressed. |
| • Father has a history of seeking mental health services for his children and responds well in crisis situations. | • Family is socially isolated, low finances. |
| | • Father exhibits low frustration tolerance, poor problem-solving and disciplinary skills. |
| | • Older sister has primary parenting responsibilities and appears depressed. |
| | • Younger brother exhibits ADHD symptoms. |
| **Peers** | |
| • B mixes well with different peer groups at school. | • B has a few older peers who have been involved in antisocial behavior at school (i.e., suspended). |
| • B has several prosocial friends in his community. | |
| • Deviant peers do not seem to be central to his problems. | |
| **School** | |
| • Father receives a lot of support from B's teacher. | • None identified. |
| • Father and teacher have a good working alliance. | |
| • Teacher is very skilled in managing behaviorally disordered adolescents and provides a very structured classroom setting with clear and unambiguous rules that are consistently enforced. | |
| **Community** | |
| • The family lives in a safe community. | • Some antisocial older boys live in the neighborhood. |

**FIGURE 7.3.** Systemic strengths and needs: Brent.

school, he exhibited volitional control and fair emotional and behavioral regulation of impulsive and aggressive behavior. At home, in contrast, Brent was easily angered and adopted a strong, hostile, and competitive stance in the family, especially toward his sister. When asked about the discrepancy in his behavior at home and at school, Brent reported that at home he was bored, that his father treated him unfairly, and that when he was frustrated with his father or sister, he became more irritable and had hostile and angry thoughts.

The father was providing for his family's basic needs, but at a significant cost to his own psychosocial functioning. The constant pressure of his financial responsibilities as a single wage earner, coupled with the emotional stress of raising a difficult child, affected his mood and energy and taxed his ability to cope. The father described having low frustration tolerance and feelings of isolation, fatigue, hopelessness in disciplining his children, and despondency when thinking about his many obligations. The father frequently ruminated about these issues, and he acknowledged that the feelings of despondency contributed to his laissez-faire approach to parenting. The father had a history of depression and anxiety, for which he had received psychiatric treatment (i.e., alprazolam) and had become addicted to the medication. The addiction to alprazolam led to forged prescriptions for which he was criminally indicted. As one might expect, this mental health treatment experience made the father wary of further evaluation by members of the MST clinical team. While acknowledging that he had few social supports to help him through difficult times, he was adamant that he could handle the stress on his own.

The father also voiced concern about the behavior of his daughter and younger son. He described his daughter as easily frustrated, often tearful, and spending most of her time with her boyfriend to the exclusion of her usual school friends and activities. According to the father, these behaviors had progressively increased during the past 8 months, but he did not feel that psychiatric evaluation or treatment were warranted. The father also described having difficulty managing the youngest son's increasingly impulsive, hyperactive, and oppositional behaviors.

### Fit Assessment

The initial assessment revealed several factors that were hypothesized to either precipitate or exacerbate Brent's aggressive behavior at home (see Figure 7.4). One of the more proximal factors was the lack of paternal supervision. In turn, this factor was associated with the father's depression, his minimal social support resources, and the practical realities of raising several children with substantive needs (i.e., a daughter who is depressed, two sons who meet DSM-IV criteria for oppositional defiant disorder and ADHD) alone. The more the father worked, the fewer opportunities he had to develop friends. Thus he became more socially isolated and despondent (Principle 1). Exacerbating the situation, Brent and his siblings demonstrated more symptoms when their father was the most exhausted. This was also the time when the father was least likely to provide consequences for inappropriate behavior. Thus, he appeared to be caught in a vicious downward spiral leading to demoralization, hopelessness, and isolation—factors compounding his depressive symptoms.

Importantly, however, home observations revealed that when the father had relatively positive affect and the energy to implement contingencies with moderate consistency, Brent and his siblings were better behaved. Moreover, evaluation at school revealed that a structured classroom setting maintained Brent's appropriate behavior in this context. It seemed reasonable to hypothesize, therefore, that Brent could behave appropriately in structured settings with clear, unambiguous rules that were consistently enforced. When this positive aspect of Brent is considered along with the significant strengths demonstrated by his father (i.e., he was extremely hard-working and loved his children very much), the

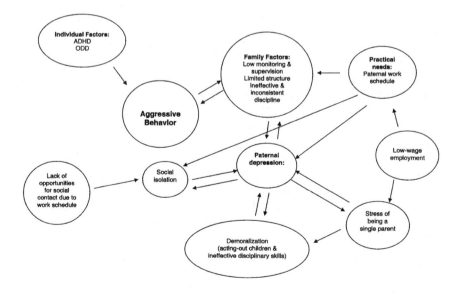

**FIGURE 7.4.** Brent's fit assessment.

understanding of fit had clear implications for the design of interventions. Likewise, verification of the diagnosis of ADHD for Brent suggested an underlying biological contributor to his behavioral difficulties for which effective pharmacological treatment is available (Barkley, 1998).

Thus, the initial assessment identified several factors directly and indirectly linked with Brent' aberrant behavior at home: (1) poor parental monitoring and ineffective discipline, (2) paternal depression, (3) social isolation, and (4) individual psychopathology (for the father, Brent, and his siblings). Consequently, with paternal buy-in, these factors became the targets of treatment.

## Overarching Goals

Family, teacher, and therapist consensus on the overarching goals for treatment were (1) eliminating Brent's physical and verbal aggression toward members of his family; (2) improving parental monitoring, supervision, and parenting skills (i.e., disciplinary practices); and (3) increasing social support resources for the family to attenuate the stress on the father. Improving parental supervision and discipline were hypothesized as critical to decreasing Brent's aggression; increasing social support, in turn, was viewed as critical to the sustainability of effective parenting.

## Safety

Because the emergency room evaluation was precipitated by highly aggressive behavior, the treatment team's immediate concern was ensuring the safety of Brent and his family. A crisis caseworker searched the home for weapons and other potentially dangerous contraband or medicines that might pose a risk to Brent or others. Brent, his father, and the therapist then developed a safety plan. The lack of structure after school, while the father was at work, placed Brent at considerable risk of behavioral problems. Hence, the MST team prioritized the provision of more structure during these hours. Also, like many youth diagnosed with ADHD, Brent was very sensitive to behavioral contingencies (Barkley, 2000). Thus, the safety plan called for Brent to participate in structured afterschool activities and to complete specific evening assignments (e.g., cleaning his room, completing homework, preparing for the next school day) and other chores as directed by his father. If successful, he could earn rewards and privileges (Principle 6). The older sister tracked his compliance, but was removed from the role of enforcer. To further increase monitoring and improve discipline, the father agreed to call randomly throughout the evening to check on Brent's progress and to praise his success in completing the evening protocol (Principles 2 and 6). If compliant, Brent was also rewarded tangibly by his father the next day. Alternatively, if Brent was unable to follow the evening protocol and acted aggressively or threatened to act aggressively, the MST team would be contacted immediately and Brent would be transported to the emergency room for evaluation and subsequent hospitalization if indicated. This safety plan capitalized on Brent's history of responding well to behavioral contingencies that provide immediate consequences (Barkley, 1997) and to his extreme distaste for the emergency room and hospital.

## Family Interventions

Using the father's tenacity, work ethic, and inherent desire to meet his children's needs as levers for change (Principle 2), the therapist was successful in engaging the father to focus on (1) improving his supervision and disciplinary practices, and (2) increasing his social supports from adults. The first phase of family intervention confirmed the treatment team's fit hypotheses by observing father's disciplinary practices and his management of conflict and behavioral problems. Home observations revealed a specific pattern of parent–child interactions that preceded his children's noncompliance. First, when Brent acted out, his father would attempt to redirect him or set a limit (e.g., "Stop bothering your sister," "Go to your room"), and Brent would become oppositional and refuse. His father would respond with frustration, yelling, screaming, and eventually empty threats of punishment—responses that may be reinforcing for some youth with ADHD. Another pattern was that the father would sometimes respond to Brent's oppositional behavior by bargaining with him or cajoling him into compliance. Thus, the therapist focused on helping the father develop competency in setting and enforcing clear and firm limits.

Toward this end, he was taught to calmly give commands that were short and to the point, provide one directive at a time, and use when–then commands that clearly specified the desired behavior he wanted from Brent and his siblings (Webster-Stratton & Herbert, 1994; Principles 3, 4, 5, 6, and 7). In addition, the father learned to give more immediate feedback and consequences, and to "act, don't yak" (Barkley, 2000). Unfortunately, as with most youth whose parents place their children's problem behavior under extinction, Brent's aggression escalated when the father began setting and enforcing limits.

Because Brent's behavior had previously escalated to physical aggression and he was physically small, his father was taught a physical hold technique called a basket-hold (Principle 6). While the father had the physical strength to hold Brent, he at times did not have the energy.

To help the father provide for Brent's safety, the therapist focused on two additional areas: (1) identifying and obtaining social supports to help manage Brent, and (2) increasing the father's energy level by decreasing his symptoms of depression (Principle 3, 4, and 9). Due to the lengthy process of finding social supports and addressing barriers to their utilization, the therapist arranged for a MST crisis caseworker to help the father manage Brent in the short term. Given the ecological focus of MST, interventions staffed by the clinical team are deemed a temporary solution until indigenous supports can be arranged. Fortunately, team support for monitoring was only necessary during the first week of treatment. The need for social supports that the father could tap during difficult times, however, remained an issue.

### Social Supports

When Brent's behavior was under better control, the broader systemic problem of the father's social isolation was addressed (Principle 9). Because the isolation was due, in part, to his work schedule, the therapist helped the father access a better paying job that would allow him to be home in the evening. Concomitantly, to increase his social contacts, the father was encouraged to attend an area church; subsequently, he joined the church's softball team. In addition, he joined a "Tough Love" parental support group available within his community. Yet these social opportunities were not sufficient to meet the father's need for instrumental assistance with parenting and emotional and appraisal support. The father was too depressed and overwhelmed with his own problems to develop sustainable social relations. Thus, the therapist hypothesized that the father's symptoms of depression needed to be treated before he could take full advantage of these newfound resources.

### Individual and Pharmacological Interventions

Depression was a major barrier to the father's completion of behavioral interventions as well as those designed to increase his social supports. Ameliorating the depression, therefore, became a target of treatment (Principle 8). Although initially reluctant to be evaluated, the father was finally convinced by the therapist to obtain an assessment by the MST psychiatrist. The assessment revealed significant neurovegetative symptoms of depression (e.g., low energy, anhedonia, appetite and sleep disturbance, poor concentration) and emotional lability (e.g., irritability, poor frustration tolerance). The psychiatrist started the father on an SSRI antidepressant. This medication trial was coupled with cognitive-behavioral interventions by the MST therapist because the father's depressive symptoms were also cognitively mediated (e.g., perseveration on negative life events).

Although the father made significant strides in following behavioral interventions, Brent's behavior remained sufficiently aberrant to warrant further psychiatric involvement (Principle 8). Using evidence-based interventions as a guideline (Greenhill et al., 1996; Pliszka et al., 2000a, 2000b), the psychiatrist increased the dose of Brent's stimulant medication and discontinued the antianxiety medication prescribed during his most recent psychiatric hospitalization due to concern that it might be increasing rather than diminishing his symptoms. As expected, Brent was noncompliant with the changes in his medication regimen and often tested limits around taking them. The father, however, used his new skills in setting limits and developing behavioral contingencies to address this problem (Principle 9). After several weeks, despite medication compliance and a decrease in ADHD symptoms based on teacher reports on a standardized measure (i.e., Conners Teacher Rating Scale; Conners, Sitarenios, Parker, & Epstein, 1998), Brent continued to complain of intense anger and frustration, sleep and appetite disturbance, and occasional sadness. Thus, he was reevaluated, and an SSRI antidepressant was combined with his stimulant medication. After approximately 3 weeks on this regimen, his symptoms of depression were significantly improved as evidenced by a decreased score on the Children's Depression Inventory (Kovacs, 1992).

While working with Brent and his father, the therapist discovered that Brent's sister, Angela, was also experiencing significant levels of depression. Because Angela's mental health status significantly impacted the well-being of the client and his father, the therapist felt that it was important to help her attain treatment as well. Subsequently, an evaluation by the MST psychiatrist confirmed a diagnosis of depression. Angela described having a profound sense of hopelessness, low frustration tolerance, crying spells, and sleep and appetite disturbances. The sister acknowledged that these symptoms were exacerbated by her responsibilities of caring for her younger siblings. Thus, Angela was also started on an SSRI antidepressant and family interventions were put into place to create more developmentally appropriate roles between Angela, her father, and siblings (Principle 6). Initially, the MST therapist attempted to provide cognitive behavioral therapy for Angela. She refused, asking for a female therapist. As this request seemed reasonable, a female MST therapist provided these interventions for several weeks.

## Outcomes

The initial safety plan and behavioral interventions eliminated Brent's physical aggression at home by the end of the first week of treatment.

During that week, Brent required a crisis caseworker in the home to help manage his aggressive behavior via contingency management and therapeutic holds, plus the threat of hospitalization. This initial crisis plan had minimal ecological validity and would fail to promote treatment generalization and maintenance (Principle 9). Nevertheless, the plan was an effective short-term solution for managing Brent's aggressive behavior until his father could develop the skills and resources needed to independently deal with this difficulty.

As with many hard-working single parents, especially those with children presenting serious emotional disturbance, the father felt demoralized and quickly learned to depend upon members of the MST treatment team to manage his children's behavior. This dependence on the MST team was evidenced by his daily calls to the therapist and crisis caseworker to intervene with his children. However, as the father improved his ability to set limits and to apply consistent consequences (Principles 4 and 5), and as the interventions addressed barriers to appropriate parenting (e.g., work schedule, depression, social isolation), the frequency of telephone calls decreased substantially. In addition, as the father felt more energized and comfortable managing his family, he became less dependent on others (e.g., MST staff, members of his new social support network; Principle 9), and was better able to follow through on the behavioral interventions that had been put into place. The father's increased parenting skills, improved access to social supports, and better paying job (with fewer hours) made him more available to be involved in his daughter's life. Concomitantly, the daughter's affect improved, and individual therapy was no longer necessary.

Brent's case highlights that for some youth experiencing a psychiatric emergency, ecological changes alone may be insufficient in managing the child's behavior. Here, developing parenting skills and indigenous social supports helped, but were insufficient to eliminate or manage all of Brent's aberrant behaviors at home, especially those that were biologically influenced (e.g., ADHD, depression). Following the appropriate maximization of stimulant and antidepressant medication, Brent's behavior at home reached subclinical levels. While he continued to test limits and his father's resolve, his behavior was less aversive to his family and more easily managed, especially after his father received appropriate psychiatric care.

## STACEY

Stacey's case illustrates the interconnections between biologically driven problems, disturbances in family transactions, the potential for siblings to exacerbate difficulties, and the role of peers in fostering problem behavior. Integrated psychoeducational, pharmacological, and family-based interventions were critical to improving outcomes for several family members.

## Presenting Information

Stacey was a 15-year-old African American female referred for psychiatric hospitalization by a mobile psychiatry crisis team following suicidal threats. Accompanying Stacey to the intake assessment were her aunt and uncle, her adoptive parents. Although Stacey had a significant history of running away (i.e., more than 10 episodes lasting from 3 to 7 days), alcohol and marijuana abuse, and physical aggression, this was her first psychiatric referral. During the intake assessment, the aunt expressed concern that Stacey's behavior had become increasingly more difficult to manage. For example, the caregivers had to nail shut windows throughout the house to prevent Stacey from leaving during the night. The aunt also reported using the police to locate Stacey after she ran away and to arrest her when she became verbally and physically aggressive toward her uncle. Stacey acknowledged that her behavior was inappropriate and becoming more severe over time. She denied current or past suicidal ideation or behavior but described homicidal ideation toward her uncle when in the midst of family arguments. Stacey reported that she hated living at home because of family conflict, but refused to elaborate further. The uncle agreed with Stacey's assessment of family life, stating that their home had become increasingly intolerable because of conflict and Stacey's disrespectful behavior toward him.

## Intake Assessment and History

Stacey had a 2-year history of daily marijuana use, her drug of choice. Her initial use of marijuana, and engagement in other antisocial behavior, coincided with the release of her 17-year-old brother, Mark, from juvenile detention. Within a month of Mark's return home, Stacey began to miss school, violate her curfew, argue more with her uncle, and associate with deviant peers. Until this point, Stacey was in regular education classes, earned average grades, and did not have behavioral problems (see Figure 7.5).

The family had a significant history of mental health problems, including substance abuse, domestic violence, and suicide. Stacey's biological parents had died in a car accident when she was an infant. Subsequently, Stacey and her brother were adopted by their mother's sister and her husband. The psychiatric history on their father's side of the family

| STRENGTHS | NEEDS |
|---|---|

### Individual

| | |
|---|---|
| • Average intelligence and insightful. | • Daily marijuana use. |
| • Cooperative with the safety plan. | • High risk for running away. |
| • Extroverted and sociable. | • Negative affective bond with caregivers. |
| • Loves animals. | • School truancy. |
| | • Impulsive. |
| | • Engages in high-risk sexual behavior when on runaway status. |
| | • Violent toward uncle. |

### Family

| | |
|---|---|
| • Family invested in helping S be successful. | • Poor affective bond between S and her uncle. |
| • Family has a history of using outside resources to help manage S. | • High conflict in home. |
| • Caregivers set limits with Mark. | • Uncle has a labile mood and memory problems as a result of a head injury. |
| • Stable marriage. | • Caregivers use poor judgment in trying to manage S's behavior. |
| • Older brother cares a great deal about S and wants the best for her. | • Brother engages in antisocial behavior and has a negative influence on S. |

### Peers

| | |
|---|---|
| • Some prosocial friends in the community and at school that have histories of regular school attendance and good grades. | • S's only close friends are associated with her older brother, and these friends encourage deviant behavior. |

### School

| | |
|---|---|
| • Recent attendance and compliance. | • S is failing the ninth grade. |
| • S has a positive relationship with the principal. | • S has been truant more days than not. |
| | • S uses drugs at school. |

### Community

| | |
|---|---|
| • The family lives in a safe community. | • Brother lives with friends in the area. |
| • Some prosocial activities and potential prosocial friends are nearby. | • Negative peers live in their community. |

**FIGURE 7.5.** Systemic strengths and needs: Stacey.

was not known. Their mother had a history of depression and substance abuse. Their uncle (adoptive father) had a history of alcohol abuse, but had been abstinent for 2 years. He also had a history of a brain injury, 4 years earlier, which resulted in difficulties with speech, memory, and mood regulation. These mental health problems had been treated extensively at the local medical center with psychotropic medications, with some efficacy according to the aunt. The uncle had discontinued these treatments several years ago while gaining sobriety through Alcoholics Anonymous. Domestic violence had occurred between Stacey's uncle and brother, and was one of several factors associated with the brother's incarceration. Finally, a maternal aunt had committed suicide.

## Safety

Safety was a significant concern during the first week of treatment. Stacey's history of running away and engaging in high-risk behaviors (e.g., unprotected sex with adult males, association with deviant peers, substance abuse), escalating violence at home, and her recent suicide threat suggested considerable risk if she returned home immediately. Thus, the team and family decided on a 2- to 3-day hospitalization to (1) comprehensively evaluate Stacey psychiatrically, (2) further assess the home environment, and (3) identify individuals and places that harbored Stacey when she ran away. Completing this latter process was a requirement of Stacey's release from the hospital. As part of the safety plan, upon release from the hospital, Stacey was monitored 24 hours a day by a combination of team and family members for purposes of crisis stabilization and direct observation of family interactions. Given that conflict between Stacey and her uncle hastened the psychiatric emergency, the safety plan also called for the uncle to temporarily allow the aunt to provide all parenting. The final element of the safety plan was a "No Harm Contract" that all family members signed. The contract detailed protocols for each family member in responding to conflict.

## Fit Assessment

The identified problems were linked with an array of factors at biological, cognitive, family relational, and peer levels (see Figure 7.6).

### FAMILY INTERACTION SEQUENCES

A good starting place for assessing youth who run away is to ask, "Is this youth running away *from* something or *to* something?" Conflict between Stacey and her uncle was the most proximal fit factor associated with running away. A clear precipitant to each episode was intense arguing between Stacey and her uncle, which often followed the uncle's attempts to set limits. According to the aunt, whenever her husband attempted to discipline Stacey (e.g., restricting her use of the phone because she broke curfew), Stacey would respond with oppositional behavior, and the uncle, in turn, would become angry to the point of losing control. According to Stacey, however, she was often punished twice by her uncle for the same transgression because he could not remember the previous sanction.

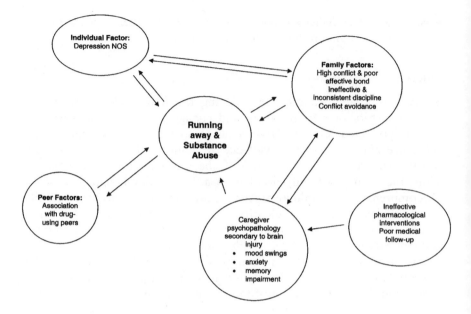

**FIGURE 7.6.** Stacey's fit assessment.

The aunt reported that during these conflicts she was placed in the arduous role of caretaker for both her husband and Stacey (i.e., calming the uncle while trying to prevent Stacey from leaving). Due to the angst generated by this sequence, the caregivers often avoided confronting Stacey or setting limits around her drug use, school attendance, and negative peer associations. Such avoidance perpetuated Stacey's deviant behavior and family stress, especially for the aunt, who often felt exhausted.

## BRAIN INJURY

Significant conflict first emerged in the family 4 years earlier following the uncle's brain injury. The family noticed that the uncle had intense mood swings; had short-term memory loss; and exhibited paranoia, panic, and generalized anxiety symptoms that often elicited negative or hostile reactions from the children. The escalating caregiver–child conflict following the brain injury eventually led to an out-of-home placement for the older brother. Mark described continued concern that his uncle and his sister may eventually harm each other.

ATTRIBUTIONAL BIASES

Home observations by the MST team revealed that Stacey often over-re-
acted to mild behavioral cues from her uncle. For example, Stacey yelled
at him one evening when he returned home and asked, "How was your
day?" When questioned about her response, Stacey replied, "He is always trying to get into my business and accuse me of stuff and start stuff
with me." Such reactions suggested that attributional bias played a role
in Stacey's emotional reactivity to her uncle. Without home observations, the reciprocal and synergistic interplay of Stacey's emotional reactivity coupled with caregiver pathology may not have been identified.

An individual cognitive assessment and psychiatric evaluation of
Stacey's emotional reactivity revealed that when she interacted with her
uncle she often "feels the same way I felt when he used to beat me and
my brother." Stacey reported that when her uncle first began being
"mean" he would yell at her, which initially made her feel nervous. This
anxiety, however, gave way to anger over time as the uncle became physically abusive and her aunt "did not do anything about it." From that
time forward, Stacey thought actively about "getting him back." Careful
assessment of the aunt, brother, and Stacey confirmed that the abuse had
stopped when the uncle gained sobriety 2 years earlier. Although Stacey
did not meet criteria for PTSD or any other anxiety disorder, her psychiatric evaluation revealed a depressive disorder.

PEER INFLUENCES

Stacey's drug use seemed directly related to her association with drug-
using peers, particularly her older brother and his friends. Drug use was
indirectly related to family conflict, as such conflict fueled her association with drug-using peers. In addition, Stacey noted that marijuana
seemed to dampen the sad feelings she often experienced when ruminat-
ing about her family life.

## Overarching Goals

The caregivers' primary treatment goals were to eliminate Stacey's running away and substance abuse, increase her compliance with caregiver
requests, increase school attendance and association with prosocial
peers, and decrease family conflict and association with deviant peers.
Stacey also indicated that she wanted to stay out of trouble, decrease her
substance abuse, and go to school. Reducing family conflict seemed to
be the first key to achieving these goals. Such conflict drove her running-

away behavior, which led to increased contact with her brother and his drug-using friends.

## Individual Interventions

In light of the role that the uncle's mood lability, memory loss, and anxiety related to his brain injury played in contributing to family conflict, treatment initially targeted these individual factors as precursors to decreasing family conflict (Principle 4). After obtaining the uncle's consent, the therapist and team psychiatrist consulted with the uncle's primary care physician. The primary care physician agreed to obtain a neurological consultation. Following the evaluations, the neurologist started the uncle on a mood stabilizer. The MST therapist, working with the uncle's neurologist, helped to monitor the efficacy and safety of this intervention. While the uncle's mood lability and irritability improved on this medication, he continued to have problems with memory and concentration—as would be expected based on the neurological assessment of his brain injury. Hence, the uncle's memory impairment continued to present a barrier to decreasing family stress and normalizing relations with the children.

## Family Interventions

Several family interventions were used to address the uncle's memory deficits and their impact on family relations. First, Stacey and her aunt were educated about the uncle's brain injury and its influence on his behavior. Toward this end, the MST therapist arranged a meeting between the family and the neurologist, who explained the uncle's injury and the behavioral implications of that injury for his day-to-day functioning. Second, after meeting with the neurologist, the family and the therapist developed a plan to use memory aids to optimize the uncle's functioning as a parent. A behavioral contract with clearly delineated rules and consequences for rule infractions was developed for Stacey and posted in the kitchen (Principles 3, 5, and 6) to serve as a memory cue for the uncle. Third, during family sessions the therapist worked on improving communication skills (e.g., "I" messages, active listening) between family members (Principle 4). Finally, family sessions focused on consolidating and reinforcing the executive functioning of the parental subsystem via aunt and uncle's conjoint agreement on, and consistent enforcement of, household rules (Principle 9). On occasions when the uncle's memory impairment contributed to caregiver–child conflict, the aunt reminded him of the posted rules. Stacey was given negative consequences for taking advantage of her uncle's memory impairment (Principle 3). Also, when Stacey tried to divide her aunt and uncle, they learned to refer to the posted rules and consequences without engaging in power struggles.

The family also developed strategies to address Stacey's substance use (Principles 3 and 4). Specifically, random urine screens were frequently conducted and the results were linked with predetermined reinforcers. Consistent with the CRA approach (Budney & Higgins, 1998) discussed previously, Stacey could earn one dollar for a clean urine screen; her earnings doubled for each consecutive clean screen (e.g., first clean screen was worth $1.00, second $2.00, third $4.00, etc.). Given the financial circumstances of the family, the most Stacey could earn in any week was $25.00. If, however, the result of the urine screen was positive, Stacey received no money and had to start over at a dollar. Until Stacey could demonstrate trustworthiness, operationalized as 1 month of clean screens, compliance with family rules, and association with prosocial peers, she received money vouchers instead of cash. The aunt and uncle also combined praise with the tangible rewards. Moreover, in an effort to strengthen the affective bond between Stacey and her uncle, he dispensed her rewards.

Despite significant gains in family functioning, Stacey continued to exhibit depressive symptoms that were unrelated to substance abuse, substance withdrawal, or family or social problems. These symptoms included labile mood, irritability, and decreased appetite. Following an evaluation by the MST psychiatrist, Stacey was started on a trial of bupropion, coupled with cognitive-behavioral therapy.

### Peer Interventions

As noted previously, a major correlate of Stacey's drug use was spending time with her older brother and his drug-using friends. Because the aunt and uncle, as well as the older brother, were adamant about his not returning home (i.e., he was an emancipated 17-year-old) due to his continued drug use, the family decided to limit his contact with Stacey. Several strategies were used in this regard. First, after preparing the caregivers, the therapist arranged for them to meet with Mark. In this meeting, the uncle and aunt (1) appealed to Mark's inherent strength, his love for his sister, to limit his contact with her, especially when using drugs; (2) demonstrated to Mark that the uncle was less volatile and receiving adequate treatment, as well as educated Mark about his uncle's brain injury; (3) provided opportunities for supervised visits; and (4) offered to support Mark's pursuit of his own long-term goals (Principle 2).

Second, the caregivers set limits with Stacey around unsupervised time with her brother and association with his deviant friends (Principle 3). Third, the caregivers reinforced and supported Stacey's association with prosocial peers. For example, she was allowed to use the car and received funds for engaging in prosocial activities (Principle 3). Finally, the caregivers tapped into one of Stacey's strengths, her love of animals, by arranging for her to perform community service by volunteering at an animal shelter and a wildlife park (Principle 2). The latter strategy provided the dual function of giving Stacey opportunities to meet same-age peers who were engaged in prosocial activities and limiting her amount of unstructured free time (Principle 9).

## School Interventions

Stacey had been dropped from the school roll due to excessive unexcused absences. School interventions focused on reenrolling Stacey in school and developing a monitoring plan for the aunt and uncle to track her attendance and academic functioning.

## Outcomes

Within the first 10 days of treatment, the 24-hour supervision plan was safely reduced to monitoring afterschool hours, and family conflicts were significantly reduced. Much of this early success was attributed to (1) the uncle being placed on appropriate medications that improved his mood lability, and (2) the shift in parenting roles to emphasize the aunt as primary disciplinarian. In addition, educating the family concerning the uncle's difficulties seemed to lessen their reactivity to his provocative behavior. These changes led to less family conflict, which made living at home less stressful and more enjoyable for everyone. Furthermore, reinforcing the caregivers' executive role (i.e., their conjoint responsibility for providing appropriate limits and rewards), coupled with broadening their range of disciplinary strategies, also reduced family conflict and stress (Principle 5). Finally, the caregivers' rapprochement with their nephew and support of his long-term goals was a major factor in limiting Stacey's association with deviant peers (Principle 2). By the second month of treatment, Mark, with parental support, joined Job Corps and moved 100 miles from the family home. He has maintained contact with the family, and his relationship with his uncle is vastly improved. By the end of treatment, Stacey was attending school daily, had not run away for 3 months, and, based on weekly urine screens, was abstinent from marijuana and other substances of abuse for more than 2 months.

## CONCLUSION

The cases discussed in this chapter provide a glimpse of MST treatment for children and adolescents who traditionally would have been treated in more restrictive settings. Each case represented a youth who was deemed by mental health professionals as acutely at risk of harm to self and others and in need of emergency psychiatric hospitalization. Each case also illustrated that multifaceted, individualized, and comprehensive evidence-based services can often safely ameliorate serious difficulties while maintaining the youth in his or her natural environment.

# PART III

# Outcomes, Ongoing Research, and Program Development

Chapters 8 and 9 are intended primarily for administrators, policy-makers, researchers, funders, advocates, and others interested in the development and performance of MST programs. Chapter 8 provides a succinct overview of the clinical- and service-level outcomes that MST programs have achieved and the accolades from leading reviewers and major organizations that these outcomes have earned. Such information is important in establishing the credibility of the model to local or state stakeholders. Chapter 9 provides an overview of the MST quality assurance system, which is critical to achieving the aforementioned outcomes. Funders and stakeholders versed in business performance will especially resonate to the aims and workings of this system.

# PART VII

## Curricula, Ongoing Research, and Program Development

CHAPTER 8

# MST Outcomes
# and Ongoing Research

---

This chapter provides a summary of the findings from research evaluations of MST and describes current replications of these findings and extensions of the model to other clinical populations. Commitment to rigorous evaluation and analyses is critical to the current and future viability of the model.

---

Rigorous evaluation has been fundamental to the development of MST and remains critical to the adaptation of MST for new populations and using different models of service delivery. Seven randomized clinical trials and one quasi-experimental trial have been published with youth presenting serious clinical problems and their families, and more than a dozen more are presently underway. The vast majority of these trials have been conducted in field settings in which the most challenging clinical populations have been targeted.

This chapter presents a broad overview of MST outcomes based on published trials, and then a more detailed description of outcomes pertaining specifically to mental health, violence, and substance use. Subsequent sections discuss findings from unpublished randomized trials and provide conceptual and methodological overviews of several substantive and multisite randomized trials that are currently being conducted. Finally, recommendations from the Surgeon General's National Action Agenda for Children's Mental Health (U.S. Public Health Service, 2000) are reviewed, and their pertinence to MST-related research and dissemination is noted.

## BRIEF OVERVIEW OF OUTCOMES
## FROM PUBLISHED TRIALS

As shown in Table 8.1, published MST outcome studies have included approximately 800 participating families, including one trial with inner-city delinquents (Henggeler et al., 1986), three trials with violent and chronic juvenile offenders (Borduin et al., 1995; Henggeler, Melton, Brondino, Scherer, & Hanley, 1997; Henggeler, Melton, & Smith, 1992; Henggeler, Melton, Smith, Schoenwald, & Hanley, 1993), substance-abusing or substance-dependent juvenile offenders with high rates of psychiatric comorbidity (Brown, Henggeler, Schoenwald, Brondino, & Pickrel, 1999; Henggeler, Clingempeel, Brondino, & Pickrel, in press; Henggeler, Pickrel, & Brondino, 1999; Schoenwald, Ward, Henggeler, Pickrel, & Patel, 1996), youths presenting psychiatric emergencies (e.g., suicidal, homicidal, psychotic) (Henggeler, Rowland, et al., 1999; Schoenwald et al., 2000), maltreating families (Brunk, Henggeler, & Whelan, 1987), and juvenile sexual offenders (Borduin, Henggeler, Blaske, & Stein, 1990). Most of the studies focused on youths who were truly at imminent risk for out-of-home placements such as incarceration, residential treatment, or psychiatric hospitalization.

Across studies, consistent clinical- and service-level outcomes have emerged. At the clinical level, in comparison with control groups, MST:

- Improved family relations and functioning.
- Increased school attendance.
- Decreased adolescent psychiatric symptoms.
- Decreased adolescent substance use.
- Decreased long-term rates of rearrest ranging from 25–70%.

At the service level and in comparison with control groups, MST has achieved:

- 97% and 98% rates of treatment completion in recent studies.
- Decreased long-term rates of days in out-of-home placement ranging from 47–64%.

## TABLE 8.1. Published MST Outcome Studies

| Study | Population | Comparison | Follow-up | MST outcomes |
|---|---|---|---|---|
| Henggeler et al. (1986) N = 57[a] | Delinquents | Diversion services | None | Improved family relations Decreased behavior problems Decreased association with deviant peers |
| Brunk, Henggeler, & Whelan (1987) N = 33 | Maltreating families | Behavioral parent training | None | Improved parent–child interactions |
| Borduin, Henggeler, Blaske, & Stein (1990) N = 16 | Adolescent sexual offenders | Individual counseling | 3 years | Reduced sexual offending Reduced other criminal offending |
| Henggeler et al. (1991)[b] | Serious juvenile offenders | Individual counseling Usual community services | 3 years | Reduced alcohol and marijuana use Decreased drug-related arrests |
| Henggeler, Melton, & Smith (1992) N = 84 | Violent and chronic juvenile offenders | Usual community services | 59 weeks | Improved family relations Improved peer relations Decreased recidivism (43%) Decreased out-of-home placement (64%) |
| Henggeler et al. (1993) | Same sample | | 2.4 years | Decreased recidivism (doubled survival rate) |
| Borduin et al. (1995) N = 176 | Violent and chronic juvenile offenders | Individual counseling | 4 years (10-year outcomes forthcoming) | Improved family relations Decreased psychiatric symptomatology Decreased recidivism (69%) |
| Henggeler, Melton, et al. (1997) N = 155 | Violent and chronic juvenile offenders | Juvenile probation services | 1.7 years | Decreased psychiatric symptomatology Decreased days in out-of-home placement (50%) Decreased recidivism (26%, nonsignificant) Treatment adherence linked with long-term outcomes |
| Henggeler, Rowland, et al. (1999) N = 116 (Final sample = 156) | Youths presenting psychiatric emergencies | Psychiatric hospitaliza-tion | None (2-year outcomes forthcoming) | Decreased externalizing problems (CBCL) Improved family relations Increased school attendance Higher consumer satisfaction |

(*continued*)

**TABLE 8.1.** (*continued*)

| Study | Population | Comparison | Follow-up | MST outcomes |
|---|---|---|---|---|
| Schoenwald et al. (2000) | Same sample | | | 75% reduction in days hospitalized<br>50% reduction in days in other out-of-home placements |
| Henggeler, Pickrel, & Brondino (1999) (*N* = 118) | Substance-abusing and substance-dependent delinquents | Usual community services | 1 year | Decreased drug use at posttreatment<br>Decreased days in out-of-home placement (50%)<br>Decreased recidivism (26% nonsignificant)<br>Treatment adherence linked with decreased drug use |
| Schoenwald et. al. (1996) | Same sample | | 1 year | Incremental cost of MST nearly offset by between-groups differences in out-of-home placement |
| Brown et al. (1999) | Same sample | | 6 months | Increased attendance in regular school settings |
| Henggeler et al. (in press) | Same sample | | 4 years | Decreased violent crime<br>Increased marijuana abstinence |

[a]Quasi-experimental design (groups matched on demographic characteristics); all other studies are randomized.
[b]Based on participants in Henggeler et al. (1992) and Borduin et al. (1995).

- Higher consumer satisfaction.
- Considerable cost savings—for example, the Washington State Institute on Public Policy (Aos, Phipps, Barnoski, & Lieb, 1999) concluded that MST produced more than $60,000 in savings per youth.

## DETAILED REVIEW OF OUTCOMES FROM PUBLISHED TRIALS

Youths with serious emotional disturbance, especially those at imminent risk of out-of-home placement, typically present a mix of serious clinical problems that can be subdivided into mental health problems, violence, and substance abuse.

### Mental Health Outcomes

The mental health report of the U.S. Surgeon General (DHHS, 1999) devoted considerable attention to MST outcomes. Reviewers (e.g., Burns et al., 1999; Kazdin & Weisz, 1998) have noted the promise of MST in treating serious mental health problems in children and adolescents. This section summarizes published mental health outcomes for children and families, and presents findings from the recent study that focused on youths presenting psychiatric emergencies.

## YOUTH EMOTIONAL AND BEHAVIOR PROBLEMS

The first published MST outcome study (Henggeler et al., 1986) showed that MST decreased the conduct problems, anxious-withdrawn behaviors, and immaturity of inner-city delinquents in comparison with counterparts receiving a variety of alternative community treatments. These findings were replicated by Borduin et al. (1995) in a study with violent and chronic juvenile offenders. In another study with violent and chronic juvenile offenders (Henggeler, Melton, et al., 1997), MST produced decreased psychiatric distress in comparison with the usual juvenile justice services.

## FAMILY FUNCTIONING

MST has consistently produced improvements in family functioning across outcome studies with juvenile offenders and maltreating families. Several of these studies used observational methods to demonstrate increased positive family interactions and decreased negative interactions (Borduin et al., 1995; Brunk et al., 1987; Henggeler et al., 1986), and others have demonstrated improved family functioning based on self-report measures (Borduin et al., 1995; Henggeler et al., 1992). In addition, significant MST effects on caregiver psychiatric symptomatology were reported by Borduin et al. (1995) and marginally significant effects were reported by Henggeler, Melton, et al. (1997).

## SCHOOL ATTENDANCE

MST effects on attendance in regular school has been evaluated in two studies. Brown et al. (1999) showed that MST improved school attendance through a 6-month follow-up in a study with substance-abusing or substance-dependent juvenile offenders. Likewise, in a study discussed next (Henggeler, Rowland, et al., 1999), MST improved the school attendance of youths who had been referred for inpatient psychiatric hospitalization because they were suicidal, homicidal, or psychotic.

## CLINICAL AND PLACEMENT OUTCOMES WITH YOUTHS PRESENTING PSYCHIATRIC EMERGENCIES

The success of MST with juvenile justice populations led to an NIMH-funded evaluation of the model as an alternative to emergency psychiatric hospitalization. Youths who were suicidal, homicidal, or psychotic were recruited from the emergency room or psychiatric inpatient admissions office after being recommended by a physician for emergency psychiatric hospitalization. Ninety percent of the families recruited agreed to participate in the study, and these youths and families ($N = 156$) were subsequently randomized to MST versus emergency psychiatric hospitalization with aftercare. If possible, the MST team (i.e., therapist, crisis caseworker, child psychiatrist) attempted to stabilize the crisis outside the hospital using the protocol described in Chapter 5. Subsequently, MST as described in Chapters 2–4 was delivered.

Short-term clinical outcomes from this study (Henggeler, Rowland, et al., 1999) show that MST was more effective than emergency hospitalization at decreasing youths' externalizing symptoms and improving their family functioning and attendance in regular school settings. MST was as effective as hospitalization at decreasing internalizing symptoms. With regard to out-of-home placements, over the first 4 months postreferral, MST produced a 72% reduction in days hospitalized and a 49% reduction in days in other out-of-home placements (Schoenwald, Ward, et al., 2000). Thus, the reduction in hospitalization was not offset by increase in other out-of-home placements. Analyses of 16-month postreferral follow-up data indicate favorable MST outcomes regarding psychiatric symptoms, family relations, and placement reduction that slowly dissipate. A manuscript describing these findings is in preparation, and an extended follow-up to 2.5 years postreferral is being conducted.

CONSUMER SATISFACTION

One study has examined consumer satisfaction with services (Henggeler, Rowland, et. al., 1999). Here, caregiver and youth satisfaction were higher for the MST condition than in the comparison condition.

## Outcomes for Criminal Behavior and Violence

As supported by the conclusions of reviewers (e.g., Farrington & Welsh, 1999; Tate et al., 1995), cited in the Surgeon General's report on youth violence (U.S. Public Health Service, 2001), and documented in Elliott's Blueprints Series (1998), MST has strong support for decreasing long-term rates of rearrest and incarceration for serious juvenile offenders.

OUTCOMES FOR REARREST AND INCARCERATION

Halliday-Boykins and Henggeler (2001) recently summarized findings from the three published randomized trials of MST with chronic and violent juvenile offenders. In the Simpsonville, South Carolina Project,

Henggeler et al. (1992) studied 84 juvenile offenders who were at imminent risk for out-of-home placement because of serious criminal activity. Youth and their families were randomly assigned to receive either MST or the usual services provided by the Department of Juvenile Justice (DJJ). At posttreatment, youth who participated in MST reported less criminal activity than their counterparts in the usual services group; at a 59-week follow-up, MST had reduced rearrests by 43%. In addition, usual services youth had an average of almost three times more weeks incarcerated (average = 16.2 weeks) than MST youth (average = 5.8 weeks). Moreover, treatment gains were maintained at long-term follow-up (Henggeler et al., 1993). At 2.4 years postreferral, twice as many MST youth had not been rearrested (39%) as usual services youth (20%).

In the Columbia, Missouri Project (Borduin et al., 1995), participants were 200 chronic juvenile offenders and their families who were referred by the local DJJ. Families were randomly assigned to receive either MST or individual therapy (IT). Four-year follow-up arrest data showed that youth who received MST were arrested less often and for less serious crimes than counterparts who received IT. Moreover, while youth who completed a full course of MST had the lowest rearrest rate (22.1%), those who received MST but prematurely dropped out of treatment had lower rates of rearrest (46.6%) than IT completers (71.4%), IT dropouts (71.4%), or treatment refusers (87.5%).

In the Multisite South Carolina Study, Henggeler, Melton, et al. (1997) examined the role of treatment fidelity in the successful dissemination of MST. In contrast with previous clinical trials in which the developers of MST provided ongoing clinical supervision and consultation (i.e., quality assurance was high), MST experts were not significantly involved in treatment implementation and quality assurance was low. Participants were 155 chronic or violent juvenile offenders who were at risk of out-of-home placement because of serious criminal involvement and their families. Youth and their families were randomly assigned to receive MST or the usual services offered by DJJ. Not surprisingly, MST treatment effect sizes were smaller than in previous studies that had greater quality assurance. Over a 1.7-year follow-up, MST reduced rearrests by 25%, which was lower than the 43% and 70% reductions in rearrest in the previous MST studies with serious juvenile offenders. Days incarcerated, however, were reduced by 47%. Importantly, high therapist adherence to the MST treatment protocols, as assessed by caregiver reports, predicted fewer rearrests and incarcerations. Thus, the modest treatment effects for rearrest in this study might be attributed to considerable variance in therapists' adherence to MST principles. As discussed in Chapter 9, these findings suggest that treatment fidelity is important in the effective dissemination of MST.

In summary, across the three trials with violent and chronic juvenile offenders, MST produced 25–70% decreases in long-term rates of rearrest, and 47–64% decreases in long-term rates of days in out-of-home placements. Significantly, more favorable outcomes were achieved under conditions of high quality assurance.

COST SAVINGS

The favorable reductions in rearrest and incarceration for MST paint a compelling picture for its cost-effectiveness. The Washington State Institute for Public Policy (1998) reviewed 16 programs for reducing juvenile crime and found MST to be the most cost-effective intervention. Moreover, a follow-up and more extensive report from this institute (Aos et al., 1999) concluded that the average net gain for MST was $61,068 per youth in criminal justice system benefits, crime victim benefits, and reduced placement costs, which contrasts, for example, with a net loss of $7,511 per youth observed for juvenile boot camps.

## Outcomes for Substance Abuse and Dependence

Reviewers have noted the promise of MST in treating substance-abusing youths (e.g., McBride et al., 1999; Stanton & Shadish, 1997). The NIDA (1999) and the Center for Substance Abuse Prevention (2001) have included MST as one of the few treatments of adolescent substance abuse with empirical support.

ENGAGEMENT AND RETENTION IN TREATMENT

Although treatment retention rates have traditionally been quite low in the area of drug treatment (Stark, 1992), MST retention in a study (Henggeler, Pickrel, & Brondino, 1999) with juvenile offenders who met formal diagnostic criteria for substance abuse (56%) or dependence (44%) was excellent. Fully 100% (58 of 58) of families in the MST condition were retained for at least 2 months of services, and 98% (57 of 58) were retained until treatment termination at approximately 4 months postreferral, averaging 40 hours of direct clinical contact with an MST therapist (Henggeler, Pickrel, Brondino, & Crouch, 1996). The effective MST family engagement strategies are described by Cunningham and Henggeler (1999).

ALCOHOL- AND DRUG-RELATED OUTCOMES

Several published clinical trials of MST have evaluated alcohol- and drug-related outcomes.

*With Serious Juvenile Offenders.* Substance-related outcomes were examined in two randomized trials of MST with violent and chronic juvenile offenders (Borduin et al., 1995; Henggeler et al., 1992), and these substance-related findings were published in a single report (Henggeler et al., 1991). Findings in the first study (Henggeler et al., 1992) showed that MST significantly reduced adolescent reports of a combined index of alcohol and marijuana use at posttreatment. In the second study (Borduin et al., 1995), substance-related arrests at a 4-year follow-up were 4% in the MST condition versus 16% in the comparison condition. In a recent meta-analysis of family-based treatments of drug abuse (Stanton & Shadish, 1997), the MST effect sizes were among the highest of those reviewed.

*With Diagnosed Substance-Abusing or Substance-Dependent Juvenile Offenders.* The effectiveness of MST was examined in a study with 118 juvenile offenders meeting DSM-III-R criteria for substance abuse or substance dependence and their families (Henggeler, Pickrel, & Brondino, 1999). Participants were randomly assigned to receive MST versus usual community services. Outcome measures assessed drug use, criminal activity, and days in out-of-home placement at posttreatment and 6-month posttreatment follow-up. Treatment adherence was examined from multiple perspectives (e.g., caregiver, youth, therapist, MST expert). MST reduced self-reported alcohol and marijuana use at posttreatment, incarceration by 46% at follow-up, and total days in out-of-home placement by 50% at follow-up. Reductions in criminal activity, however, were not as large as have been obtained previously for MST. Examination of treatment adherence measures suggested that the modest results of MST were due, at least in part, to low treatment adherence.

Nevertheless, this study provided the first demonstration of long-term treatment effects from a randomized clinical trial with substance abusing adolescents. At a 4-year follow-up (Henggeler et al., in press), results from urine screens repeated twice during 12 months showed significantly higher rates of marijuana abstinence for MST participants, 55% versus 28% of young adults. In addition, analyses demonstrated significant long-term treatment effects for aggressive criminal activity favoring MST participants, .15 versus .57 convictions per year.

## COST SAVINGS FOR SUBSTANCE-ABUSING AND SUBSTANCE-DEPENDENT JUVENILE OFFENDERS

Within the context of the randomized trial with substance-abusing or substance-dependent juvenile offenders (Henggeler, Pickrel, & Brondino, 1999), the incremental costs of MST were examined and related to observed reductions in days of incarceration, hospitalization, and residential treatment at approximately 1 year postreferral (Schoenwald et al., 1996). Results showed that the incremental costs of MST were nearly offset by the savings incurred as a result of reductions in days of out-of-home placement during the year. This study did not assess savings resulting from reduced criminal justice or crime victim costs.

## OUTCOMES FROM RECENTLY COMPLETED TRIALS OUTSIDE THE FSRC

Four additional trials of MST with serious juvenile offenders have been recently completed. Two trials were true effectiveness studies (Leschied & Cunningham, 2001; Miller, 1998), and the others (Borduin, Schaeffer, & Heiblum, 2002; Thomas, Holzer, & Wall, 2002) were conducted by university faculty with challenging community samples. With the exception of Miller (1998), outcome-related publications from these trials will be forthcoming. Miller (1998), consequently, is presented in more detail.

### Delaware Alternative to Secure Care Project

Dr. Marsha L. Miller (1998), supported by the Delaware Department of Services for Children, Youth and Their Families, examined recidivism and cost outcomes in a randomized trial ($N = 54$) of serious juvenile offenders assigned to either MST or secure care. This project began in 1995 and examined one of the first attempts to disseminate MST to community-based providers. To the credit of state decision makers, a randomized experimental design was used to evaluate the program. During the first year of the 2 years of operation, however, the MST program experienced significant implementation problems, with minimal treatment fidelity and 100% turnover of clinical staff. Nevertheless, the program subsequently stabilized.

Several key findings were reported, and these are highly pertinent to the issue of dissemination to real-world settings. First, MST recidivism during the first year was high (i.e., 67%), but was greatly reduced during the second year of operation (i.e., 35%). This reduction, in our opinion and as suggested by Miller, was most likely due to the implementation of stronger quality assurance mechanisms than were being used during the first year of operation. Indeed, anecdotal feedback from most of the first cohort of MST dissemination sites indicated that outcomes were being compromised by poor treatment fidelity. The FSRC and MST Services (Chapter 9) consequently redoubled quality assurance efforts. Across years, the recidivism rate for youths in the MST condition was the same as that for counterparts in the secure placement condition for 12 months following referral (i.e., about 50%). Hence, MST reduced rearrest when implemented with increased fidelity, but poor implementation led to increased criminal offending.

Cost-related findings were more straightforward. Offenders in the comparison condition cost an average of $25,850 per youth in placement services. In comparison, youths in the MST condition cost an average of $11,513 in MST services and an additional $5,435 in placement costs (for those MST youths subsequently placed), for a total of $16,948 per youth. Hence, MST saved $8,902 per youth in service and placement costs. The high cost for the MST services in this instance was due to the fact that the program generally operated at less than 50% of capacity, thereby inflating the cost per youth. Miller noted that low utilization was largely the product of difficulties in program implementation and interagency relations. The cost savings would have been considerably greater had the MST program served the intended number of youths and families.

## Multisite Ontario Trial

Under the direction of Dr. Alan W. Leshied (A. Cunningham, investigator), a multisite randomized trail of MST has recently been completed in Ontario, Canada. The Canadian Young Offenders Act has encouraged provincial jurisdictions to develop community-based alternatives to custody for high-risk juvenile offenders. MST was imported to address this need. Beginning in 1997, Dr. Leschied, a highly respected researcher in the field of delinquency, and his colleagues have been conducting a four-site trial of MST for high-risk youth. This is the first multisite MST trial conducted outside the FSRC, is a true effectiveness study (e.g., with real-world practitioners, quality assurance provided by MST Services), and includes the largest sample size for a completed MST trial to date. As described by Leschied and Cunningham (2001), interim results with the first 147 cases have shown that, in comparison with usual services, MST has improved family functioning, decreased recidivism by 25%, and produced cost savings. The investigators are currently examining outcomes for the full sample and examining the linkages between treatment fidelity and outcomes. Additional reports and publications from this research group can be viewed on their website, *www.lfcc.on.ca*.

## Juvenile Sexual Offender Replication

As noted previously, Borduin et al. (1990) conducted the only published randomized trial with juvenile sexual offenders in the literature. Though modest in scope (i.e., N = 16), this study supported the efficacy of MST in reducing sexual reoffending. Dr. Charles M. Borduin and his colleagues at the University of Missouri (2002) have recently replicated these findings with a sample of 48 juvenile sexual offenders randomly assigned to MST versus usual juvenile justice services. At posttreatment, compared with youths who received usual services, youths who received MST evidenced fewer behavioral problems, less criminal offending, improved peer relations, improved family relations, better grades in school, and their caregivers showed decreased psychiatric symptomatology. In addition, youths in the MST condition spent an average of 75 fewer days in out-of-home placement during the first year following referral to treatment than did youths in the usual services condition. Most importantly, an 8-year follow-up showed that youths who participated in MST were less likely than their usual services counterparts to be arrested for sexual (12.5% vs. 41.7%) and nonsexual (29.2% vs. 62.5%) crimes and spent 67% fewer days incarcerated as adults.

Currently, Dr. Borduin is collaborating with the FSRC to seek funding for a randomized effectiveness trial of MST with a larger sample of juvenile sexual offenders. The study site will be distal to the University of Missouri and the FSRC, and treatment will be delivered by community practitioners. Current MST quality assurance standards will be provided, however, to support treatment fidelity.

### The Island Youth Programs

The Island Youth Programs (Thomas et al., 2002) was a broad and comprehensive community-based approach to addressing youth violence in a distinct geographic area (i.e., Galveston Island). Directed by Dr. Christopher R. Thomas, of the University of Texas Medical Branch at Galveston, five state-of-the-art prevention, early intervention, and treatment programs were provided to area children, adolescents, and families in an integrated fashion with the support of several foundations and governmental authorities. MST was provided to those youths and families presenting the most serious antisocial behavior. As with the Delaware Secure Placement Project, Galveston represented one of the first efforts to disseminate MST to a real-world setting.

Although MST-specific outcomes have not yet been analyzed by the investigators, Thomas and his colleagues report extremely impressive findings for the five programs in their entirety. From 1994 to 1998, the duration of the project, juvenile arrests for violent offenses in Galveston decreased by 83% (vs. a 19% reduction nationally) and total juvenile arrests decreased by 43% (vs. a 1% increase nationally). These findings strongly support the viability of integrating evidence-based prevention and intervention models (Elliott, 1998) to impact rates of community offending.

## Summary

Recent research conducted outside the FSRC has supported the clinical and cost-effectiveness of the MST model. Importantly, differences in treatment effects between studies seem related to critical issues of treatment effectiveness and dissemination research, as discussed in Chapter 9. The differences in recidivism between Miller (1998; 0%), Leschied and Cunningham (2001; 25%), and Borduin et al. (2002; 53%) are similar to the differences observed between Henggeler, Melton, et al. (1997), Henggeler et al. (1992), and Borduin et al. (1995). Henggeler, Melton, et al. (1997) was conducted in community mental health centers, and did not have strong quality assurance (25% reduction in rearrest). Henggeler et al. (1992) was also conducted in a community mental health center, but one of the developers of MST provided ongoing clinical consultation (43% reduction in rearrest). In contrast, Borduin et al. (1995) was conducted in a university setting, supervised closely by an MST developer, and had the largest effect sizes (70% reduction in rearrest). These findings, in conjunction with research discussed subsequently linking MST adherence to youth and family outcomes (e.g., Huey et al., 2000), further reinforce the importance of providing an ongoing focus on treatment fidelity in MST programs.

## ONGOING RANDOMIZED TRIALS, QUASI-EXPERIMENTAL STUDIES, AND ADAPTATIONS OF MST

This section addresses MST studies conducted by investigators at the FSRC and by universities and state authorities.

### Ongoing Studies under the Direction of FSRC Investigators

The FSRC is conducting several randomized trials and two quasi-experimental studies aimed at expanding the scope of MST interventions in several directions: enhancing the effectiveness of the model, adapting the model for use with different clinical populations, providing services in different contexts, and using different models of service delivery.

#### YOUTHS WITH SERIOUS EMOTIONAL DISTURBANCE

A recently completed study, directed by Rowland and her colleagues (Rowland et al., 2002), examined the short-term clinical and placement outcomes for 31 youth with serious emotional disturbance at imminent risk of placement. Adolescents approved for out-of-home placement were randomly assigned to intensive MST treatment or Hawaii's existing continuum of care. Assessments examining symptomatology, antisocial behavior, substance use, family functioning, school placement, and out-of-home placement were conducted at intake and 6-months post-referral. Largely replicating the findings for MST as an alternative to emergency psychiatric hospitalization, results showed that MST youth experienced significant reductions in externalizing symptoms, dangerousness to self or others, and days in out-of-home placement (75% decrease). Trends favoring MST were observed for decreased criminal activity, time in regular school settings (66% increase), and improved caregiver satisfaction with social supports. Although the small sample size and corresponding low statistical power mitigate firm conclusions regarding treatment effects, this randomized trial further supports the use of MST with youth experiencing significant psychiatric symptoms and provides the first outcome data supporting the use of MST with youth primarily of Asian ethnicity.

## PHYSICALLY ABUSED CHILDREN AND ADOLESCENTS

Child physical abuse carries significant short- and long-term consequences for children and families and costs to society. A large body of literature supports a multidetermined etiology of maltreatment, yet most treatment approaches address single factors and evidence of treatment effectiveness is limited (Becker et al., 1995). To address these difficulties, Dr. Cynthia Cupit Swenson has been funded by the NIMH to conduct a randomized trial of MST versus group behavioral parent training in treating physically abused children and adolescents and their families. This study builds on one of the few randomized trials in the child maltreatment literature: an MST study directed by Dr. Molly Brunk and her colleagues (Brunk et al., 1987) that achieved reasonably strong outcomes, but was limited in scope and included no follow-up. Swenson's project is an effectiveness trial (e.g., therapists are practitioners working in a community mental health center) and will eventually include 214 families with an "indicated" case of physical abuse against a child. Measures are examining child, parent, family, and service system (e.g., reincidence of maltreatment, cost) outcomes; a 12-month follow-up is included. Thus, the study will determine whether MST attenuates the negative outcomes that abused children experience and parental abusive behavior in a cost-effective fashion.

## JUVENILE DRUG COURT

Juvenile drug courts have two basic components: (1) frequent (e.g., weekly) appearances before the judge during which he or she reviews the offender's use of drugs through urine drug screens, and then applies rewards or sanctions based on the results; and (2) referral to and monitoring of compliance with community-based substance abuse treatment. Although juvenile drug courts hold potential for improving the outcomes of juvenile offenders with substance abuse problems, these courts are being disseminated across the nation with little empirical support, and the vast majority use substance abuse treatment models with no empirical support (Belenko, 1998). In collaboration with the Charleston Drug Court and juvenile justice authorities, the FSRC (Henggeler, principal investigator; Drs. Cunningham, Halliday-Boykins, and Randall, investigators) is conducting a four-group randomized trial funded by the NIDA and the NIAAA. The study will eventually include 288 juvenile offenders meeting diagnostic criteria for substance abuse or substance dependence; outcomes assessed through an 18-month follow-up pertain to drug use, criminal behavior, psychiatric functioning, family functioning, peer and school relations, service utilization, and cost-effectiveness.

The study addresses several important issues. First, does the relatively intensive juvenile drug court produce better clinical and service outcomes than family court, where youths are seen once every 6 months? Here, youths receiving drug court and usual community substance abuse services are compared with youths receiving family court and usual community substance abuse services. Second, does the addition of an evidence-based substance abuse treatment (i.e., MST) to juvenile drug court improve outcomes versus juvenile drug court with usual community substance abuse services? Third, does the integration of components of the CRA model (Budney & Higgins, 1998) to standard MST improve MST outcomes? Our expectations are that MST will enhance drug court outcomes and that the integration of CRA components will improve the ability of MST to achieve substance-related outcomes.

## MST-BASED CONTINUUM OF CARE

As described in Chapter 6, a randomized trial of an MST-based continuum of care is being conducted in Philadelphia (Dr. Schoenwald, principal investigator; Drs. Henggeler, Letourneau, Randall, and Rowland, investigators). The goal of the study is to demonstrate that evidence-based continua of care can achieve superior clinical outcomes at significant cost savings, with the hope that such savings can be used to support evidence-based prevention and early intervention programs. The study will eventually include 200 youths with serious emotional disturbance randomly assigned to the MST continuum versus usual intensive mental health services (typically, an out-of-home placement). The project is a collaboration between the City of Philadelphia mental health and juvenile justice authorities and focuses on serious juvenile offenders who present significant mental health problems and would otherwise be placed in residential facilities. Outcomes focus on mental health, drug use, criminal activity, family functioning, school functioning, and service utilization.

## NEIGHBORHOOD SOLUTIONS FOR NEIGHBORHOOD PROBLEMS

This quasi-experimental neighborhood-level intervention project (Randall, Swenson, & Henggeler, 1999; Dr. Swenson, principal investigator) examines the degree to which a neighborhood can be empowered through the provision of evidence-based services to address problems identified by neighborhood residents. The neighborhood was selected based on its rates of poverty, unemployment, child maltreatment, arrests, and school problems; it had some of the highest rates of these factors in the state of South Carolina. Neighborhood residents and stakeholders identified adolescent drug dealing, adolescent drug abuse, child prostitution, and school expulsion and suspension as the most pressing child- and family-related problems in the neighborhood. With community collaboration, interventions were designed to address these issues. A comparison neighborhood with similar demographics is being used to evaluate possible cost savings and reductions in identified problems. This study will inform the ways in which evidence-based mental health services can be used to attenuate the deleterious effects of neighborhood disadvantage on child and family outcomes.

## HEALTHY CHILDREN THROUGH HEALTHY SCHOOLS

Cunningham and Henggeler (2001; Dr. Cunningham, principal investigator) are conducting a quasi-experimental study of evidence-based prevention and interventions at the school level. Two middle schools were selected that serve predominantly African American and economically disadvantaged children and that have high rates of violence, drug use, and dropout. A mental health team is implementing empirically based violence and drug abuse prevention programs for the entire student body and providing consultation to teachers. In addition, MST is provided to youth who have been expelled, have been found with drugs, or have perpetrated crimes in school. One school initially served as a comparison while the intervention was implemented at the other school. Subsequently, interventions are being conducted at both schools. Reductions in emotional and behavioral problems and cost savings are the key outcomes that will be examined. Findings will have implications for the development of school-based prevention programs and mental health services.

TRANSPORTABILITY STUDY

Dr. Sonja K. Schoenwald is the principal investigator of an NIMH-funded study examining the effective transport of MST to community settings. As noted previously, MST has been identified by the NIMH, the NIDA, the CSAP, and the Office of Juvenile Justice and Delinquency Prevention as an effective treatment model that should be disseminated to community-based service providers. Such transport, however, has presented many challenges at multiple levels (Schoenwald & Henggeler, 2002), including factors associated with therapist, supervisor, agency, and interagency contexts. Because therapist adherence to MST is crucial to obtaining favorable outcomes, this complex study is modeling therapist adherence and family outcomes from a well-conceived set of predictor variables across practitioner, agency, and community systems. The study includes consumers and service providers at 41 sites currently implementing MST in the United States and Canada. Participants will include 2,550 youth and families referred to MST programs, as well as the clinicians and administrators employed by these programs. Not only will this study help in understanding the key elements to the effective dissemination of MST, but it will also inform efforts to disseminate other types of evidence-based treatments to community settings.

## Ongoing Studies under the Direction of Investigators Outside the FSRC

Several multisite studies of MST with juvenile offenders are in progress, and others projects are examining the adaptation of MST for treating different clinical populations.

### NORWEGIAN MULTISITE CLINICAL TRIAL

Directed by Dr. Terje Ogden, at the University of Oslo, an MST effectiveness trial is being conducted across four of the 17 sites in Norway that have formal MST programs. Interestingly, Norway has little tradition for evaluating treatment programs, and this project was the first of its kind in the country. Participants will eventually include 100 youths referred for serious behavior problems such as criminal offenses and substance abuse and their families. Youths and families are assigned randomly to either MST or usual services conditions, and outcome evaluations are conducted at 6-month intervals through 18 months post-referral. Outcome measures pertain to youth mental health, criminal activity, and substance use; family relations; peer relations; rearrests; and out-of-home placements. Treatment fidelity is being tracked and subsequent analyses will link fidelity with outcomes. In addition, key materials have been translated into Norwegian. For example, Henggeler, Schoenwald, et al. (1998) has been translated as *Multisystemisk behandling av barn og unge med atferdsproblemer*, published in Oslo by Kommuneforlaget, with a foreword by Dr. Ogden. As of early 2001, 90 adolescents and their families have already been recruited into the study. Although outcome analyses have not yet been conducted, anecdotal evidence suggests that the program is achieving its desired goals (Ogden, 2001).

## WASHINGTON STATE MULTISITE CLINICAL TRIAL

In 1997 the Washington State legislature passed the Community Juvenile Accountability Act, which provided funding for the implementation of evidence-based juvenile justice services across the state. The Washington State Institute for Public Policy was charged with identifying intervention programs with demonstrated effectiveness, and MST was supported as such. Under the direction of Drs. Robert Barnoski and Steve Aos, a quasi-experimental evaluation is being conducted with more than 100 youths and controls participating in MST programs across three sites. Preliminary 6-month recidivism results are expected in 2002, with the evaluation to be completed by June 2003 (Barnoski & Aos, personal communication, 2001). This project is noteworthy for the vision of the legislators (i.e., mandating evidence-based treatments) and the investigators (i.e., convincing the legislature to track project outcomes in a controlled fashion).

## NEW YORK MULTISITE CLINICAL TRIAL

The New York State Office of Children and Family Services, Bureau of Program Design and Resource Development, is conducting a three-site (i.e., Bronx, Queens, and Onondaga County) MST trial with Dr. Reese Satin (2000) as the principal investigator. Using a quasi-experimental design (i.e., eligible participants are referred to MST based on space availability; eligible youths for whom no space is available constitute the control group), 120 serious juvenile offenders will participate. In this study, MST is being provided as aftercare to residential placement, with the placement ending early to accommodate the MST program and allow the potential for cost savings. Outcome measures focus on recidivism and out-of-home placements, and will be collected for at least 12 months postreferral. If results are positive, the Office of Children and Family Services will consider using MST as an alternative to incarceration, which is the preferred use from our perspective. As with the Norwegian, Canadian, and Washington State projects, this New York project represents a potentially important resource and policy shift: treating serious juvenile offenders with evidence- and community-based services.

## STARK COUNTY MENTAL HEALTH BOARD, OHIO

Dr. Jane Timmons-Mitchell, at the Center for Innovative Practices, Stark County Mental Health Board, is directing two MST outcome studies (Timmons-Mitchell, personal communication, 2001). The first, funded by the Ohio Office of Criminal Justice Services, is a randomized trial of 50 juvenile offenders who were convicted of crimes and sentenced to a suspended commitment. Youths are referred either to MST delivered by a mental health agency or to usual court services, and follow-up will extend to 12 months posttreatment. Outcome measures assess youth symptomatology and functioning, rearrest, and out-of-home placements. Findings at posttreatment are supporting the capacity of MST to improve youth functioning and decrease rates of rearrest and incarceration. More extensive outcome analyses, however, will be conducted upon completion of the follow-up assessments. In addition to this randomized trial, Dr. Timmons-Mitchell is conducting a quasi-experimental study of MST with domestically violent youth referred to court. This latter study, funded by the Ohio Department of Mental Health, is the first MST study to focus specifically on domestic violence.

## VANDERBILT UNIVERSITY

The Center for Psychotherapy Research and Policy at Vanderbilt University, under the direction of Dr. Bahr Weiss, principal investigator, and Drs. Tom Catron and Vicki Harris, investigators (Weiss, Catron, & Harris, 2001), is conducting an NIMH-funded investigation of MST with 240 middle school and high school students, and their families, enrolled in classrooms designed for students with serious behavior problems. Youths are randomly assigned to treatment conditions: either MST, which prioritizes returning the youth to mainstream classrooms as a treatment goal, or continued service in the special classrooms for youth with serious emotional disturbance. The design includes a 12-month follow-up, and assessments target the individual functioning of the parent and child, family relations, peer relations, criminal activity, school functioning, and cost-effectiveness. This study is being conducted by a highly respected team of investigators, and the targeted population (i.e., youths in classrooms for behavioral problems) is unique among MST studies.

## WAYNE STATE UNIVERSITY, CHILDREN'S HOSPITAL OF MICHIGAN

This extremely innovative project, directed by Dr. Deborah A. Ellis, principal investigator, in collaboration with Drs. Sylvie Naar-King, Maureen Frey, Nancy Greger, and Cynthia Arfken (2000), and supported by the National Institute on Diabetes and Kidney Disease, is adapting MST to treat children and adolescents with insulin-dependent diabetes mellitus (IDDM) who are under poor metabolic control. Poor metabolic control is a powerful risk factor for the development of diabetes complications such as major organ failure, amputation, and premature death. Youths with poorly controlled IDDM are being randomly assigned to a pediatric adaptation of MST versus standard care. Outcome measures are examining biological indices of metabolic control, treatment adherence, family functioning, general health habits, illness management, and other constructs pertinent to pediatric care. Results from a pilot study in support of this project are very positive. This study has opened an entire new area of MST-related research. For example, investigators at other universities are developing plans to adapt MST for use with youths who have received organ transplants and are at high risk of rejection due to medication noncompliance.

## SURGEON GENERAL'S ACTION AGENDA FOR CHILDREN'S MENTAL HEALTH

As discussed in the Surgeon General's report (U.S. Public Health Service, 2000), Dr. David Satcher's conference on developing an action agenda for children's mental health was held on September 18 and 19, 2000. A broad spectrum of mental health stakeholders was included. The explicit goal of the conference was to develop a set of recommendations aimed at enhancing the nation's capacity to improve the appropriate diagnoses and treatment of children with emotional and behavioral conditions. Importantly, although the responsibility for mental health care is dispersed across several service sectors, Dr. Satcher noted that "the first system is the family, and this agenda reflects the voices of youth and family" (p. 2).

Eight broad goals are specified in the report, and each includes several action steps. Six of these goals have direct relevance to MST research and dissemination efforts. The other two (i.e., Goal 1: Promote public awareness of children's mental health issues and reduce stigma associated with mental illness; Goal 3: Improve the assessment of and recognition of mental health needs in children) are certainly pertinent, but the implications are less direct (e.g., greater public awareness of mental health needs of children entering the juvenile justice system might increase public support for treating such youths with community-based services vs. incarcerating them).

•  *Goal 2: Continue to develop, disseminate, and implement scientifically proven prevention and treatment services in the field of children's mental health.* Multiple action steps under this rubric are pertinent to MST. Examples include assessing the short- and long-term outcomes of treatment efforts; researching factors that facilitate or impede implementation and dissemination of evidence-based services; evaluating the effects of organizational and financing structures on use of evidence-based practices; developing forums among stakeholders to facilitate the adoption of evidence-based treatments; and creating a FDA-like oversight system to identify and approve scientifically based treatments.

•  *Goal 4: Eliminate racial/ethnic and socioeconomic disparities in access to mental health care services.* Interestingly, MST is the evidence-based practice that, proportionately, has probably been most accessible to minorities and the economically disadvantaged. The action steps under this rubric include increasing the accessibility of evidence-based treatments; colocating mental health treatments with other key systems such as juvenile justice and substance abuse treatment; diverting youth with mental health problems from the juvenile justice system; and conducting research on reducing health care disparities. Each of these action steps is already a central thrust of the MST delivery system or research efforts.

•  *Goal 5: Improve the infrastructure for children's mental health services, including support for scientifically proven interventions across professions.* The primary emphasis of the action steps is to create incentives and support for practitioners and agencies to use evidence-based treatments that focus on the family as the unit of change. Clearly, major barriers to the dissemination of MST are reimbursement systems that support the use of out-of-home placements by, for example, allowing providers to shift treatment costs to another agency or paying high rates to placements and low rates to community-based services. Shifting policies to emphasize the importance of families and cost-effectiveness would greatly support the dissemination of certain evidence-based practices.

•  *Goal 6: Increase access to and coordination of quality mental health care services.* Emphases of the action steps are to improve the organization of mental health services across the service sectors, enhance the role of families in treatment planning and advocacy, and develop universal systems to track outcomes. These steps fit closely with the central role that families play in the development and implementation of

MST services, as well as with continuing efforts to develop and validate continuous quality improvement systems for MST sites.

• *Goal 7: Train frontline providers to recognize and manage mental health care issues, and educate mental health providers about scientifically proven prevention and treatment services.* One of the key action steps is to require training in evidence-based practices for mental health specialists (e.g., psychiatry, psychology, social work, and nursing) and monitor the effectiveness of training efforts. Ongoing training and continuous monitoring of treatment fidelity for practitioners are already critical feature of the MST quality assurance protocol, and this system can serve as a model for other evidence-based practices.

• *Goal 8: Monitor the access to and coordination of quality mental health care services.* Key action steps include the development of national quality improvement protocols and encouragement of public and private health care organizations to ensure accountability by tracking process and outcome measures. Again, supporting the ongoing tracking of treatment fidelity and outcomes are already critical aspects of MST programs and quality assurance protocols.

## CONCLUSION

By the year 2004, more than 5,000 families will have participated in MST-related research, adaptations of the model for different clinical populations and models of service delivery will be better understood, and understanding of the parameters of effective dissemination will be advanced. Nevertheless, many research and implementation challenges must be addressed to make effective treatments readily available to children with complex problems and their families. Some of these challenges are spelled out in the Surgeon General's National Action Agenda for Children's Mental Health (U.S. Public Health Service, 2000), and characterize MST development and dissemination efforts. The authors sincerely hope that the commitment to rigorous research that has guided the development and dissemination of MST will continue to help move the field forward.

CHAPTER 9

# MST Quality Assurance
## Promoting Effective Implementation in the Field

---

This chapter describes the components of the quality assurance system used in MST programs as well as the interrelations of these components. This quality assurance system is critical to achieving the clinical- and service-level outcomes that are the overarching objectives of MST programs. Likewise, this system can serve as a model to support the fidelity of other mental health programs.

---

As community demand for MST programs increased in the mid-1990s, the challenges of implementing MST with the fidelity required to obtain positive outcomes in diverse community settings became apparent. The organizational contexts and contingencies influencing probation officers in juvenile justice settings and therapists in mental health settings are vastly different from those influencing counterparts participating in randomized clinical trials (Schoenwald & Henggeler, 2002). Indeed, experts in criminal justice (Gendreau, 1996; Gendreau & Goggin, 1997), drug abuse (Backer & David, 1995; Brown, 1995), and children's mental health (Burns et al., 1999; Kazdin & Weisz, 1998) have noted that effective transport of evidence-based interventions to real-world settings is difficult to accomplish. This section describes a quality assurance system that has been developed to support the capacity of MST programs to achieve desired clinical outcomes in community settings and presents the evidence supporting the effectiveness of this system. This quality assurance system includes ongoing training and support for MST therapists and clinical supervisors and cultivation of work environments (organizational and interagency contexts) that support the outcomes-oriented goals of MST. The quality assurance system continues to be refined in response to feedback from community-based providers and evaluation data.

The overriding purpose of the MST quality assurance system is to help therapists and supervisors achieve desired clinical outcomes for youths and families (Henggeler & Schoenwald, 1999). Figure 9.1 presents an overview of this system. The therapist's linkage with the family is viewed as primary because of its critical role in achieving outcomes (Henggeler, Schoenwald, & Munger, 1996). Several structures and processes are used to support therapist adherence to MST when interacting with families. These include *manualization* of key components of the MST program, *training* of key clinical and administrative staff in the MST program, *ongoing feedback* to the therapist from the supervisor and MST expert consultant, *objective feedback* from caregivers on a

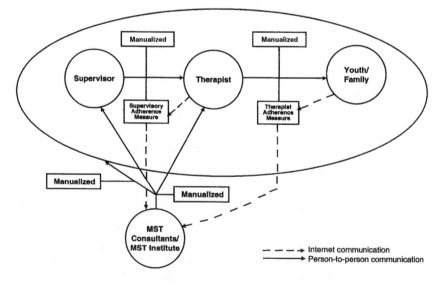

FIGURE 9.1. MST continuous quality assurance system.

standardized adherence questionnaire, and *organizational consultation.* By providing multiple layers of clinical and programmatic support and ongoing feedback from several sources, the system aims to detect deviations from fidelity quickly, identify factors contributing to these deviations, and implement strategies needed to enhance fidelity.

## MANUALIZATION OF PROGRAM COMPONENTS

The manualization of clinical, supervisory, consultative, and administrative procedures has formed the basis for the standardization of MST programs. Data from clinical trials clearly show that youth outcomes are more favorable when MST is implemented with high integrity. In light of the great diversity of children and families served by MST programs, as well as of the practitioners and staff working in MST programs, structures and processes are needed to focus stakeholders on the ultimate goals of MST programs: decreasing out-of-home placements, decreasing behaviors that lead to placement, and enhancing youth and family functioning. The following manuals play important roles in providing such structure and delineating the playing field of MST programs.

### Treatment

An earlier volume on MST interventions for youth with serious antisocial behavior (Henggeler et al., 1998) has served as a treatment manual for clinicians in MST programs in community-based settings. The present book specifies in detail the MST approach to the treatment of youths with serious emotional disturbances and their families.

### Supervision

The overarching objective of MST supervision is to facilitate therapists' acquisition and implementation of the conceptual and behavioral skills required to adhere to the MST treatment model. As such, supervision serves three interrelated purposes: (1) development of case-specific recommendations to speed progress toward outcomes for each client family, (2) monitoring of therapist adherence to MST treatment principles in all cases, and (3) advancement of clinicians along their developmental trajectories with respect to each aspect of the ongoing MST assessment and intervention process. Just as therapists are encouraged to "do whatever it takes" to achieve treatment goals with families, supervisors must be prepared to expend considerable effort in promoting clinicians' adherence to the MST protocol. The MST supervisory manual (Henggeler

& Schoenwald, 1998) is structured to orient supervisors to processes that are important to the success of MST supervision, therapist adherence, and child/family outcomes. In addition, the manual includes sections aimed at resolving difficulties that arise during supervision and barriers that arise in the treatment of families.

MST supervision has several key features. First, because seasoned clinicians are typically accustomed to practicing independently, they often perceive compulsory supervision as a foreign experience when they begin to work with MST programs. Several assumptions about MST supervision are explicitly discussed to help clinicians embrace active supervision of their cases as necessary and supportive of their work. These assumptions reflect respect for therapists as competent professionals, the compatibility of supervision with such professionalism, and the parallel processes of MST treatment and supervision.

Second, MST supervision typically occurs in a group format. Three–four therapists and their supervisor meet together at least once each week, for 1.5–2 hours per session. Supervision sessions may occur two or more times weekly when clinicians and supervisors are new to MST, and three times per week when MST is used as an alternative to psychiatric hospitalization for youth in crises. Indeed, daily supervision may be needed when crisis stabilization plans are activated. In addition, all supervisors conduct periodic field supervision and reviews of therapists' audiotaped treatment sessions to ensure that they have continued firsthand experience with clinician performance in the field. Therapists prepare summaries of each case for supervision (as described earlier) and supervisors develop, note, and update recommendations for each case.

Third, since few clinicians possess all clinical competencies required to execute MST, on-site supervisors, usually in collaboration with MST consultants, provide training experiences (e.g., appropriate reading, role-played exercises, etc.) to assist with the development of needed skills (e.g., marital interventions, cognitive-behavioral interventions for depressed adults, etc.). When the requisite skills exist, but evidence from weekly supervision and adherence measures suggests that a particular clinician is not adhering to MST principles and is making little progress in most of his or her cases, individual supervision may be warranted. The purpose of such individual sessions is for the supervisor and the therapist to jointly assess the fit of the lack of adherence and poor progress and then to develop strategies to remedy the situation. Factors contributing to poor adherence can include case-specific dilemmas, supervisor behavior, and therapist factors, and strategies for assessing and addressing each are presented in the supervision manual.

## Expert Consultation

As specified in a consultation manual (Schoenwald, 1998) and depicted in Figure 9.1, an MST expert plays an important role as a consultant who teaches clinicians and supervisors how to implement MST effectively and how to identify and address organizational and systemic barriers to program success. Consultants are expected to be highly knowledgeable regarding the theoretical and empirical underpinnings of MST as well as the use of evidence-based child and adolescent treatments and mental health services research. Through weekly phone consultations and quarterly on-site booster sessions with therapists and supervisors, the consultant provides ongoing evaluation and feedback regarding the team's implementation of MST. In addition, considerable attention is devoted to developing the skills of the on-site supervisors. The consultant is also responsible for helping the team and the organization overcome internal and external barriers to successful implementation of MST.

## Organizational Support

The MST organizational manual (Strother et al., 1998) is a resource for administrators of organizations developing MST programs. The manual provides an introduction to the theory and practice of MST and describes particular areas of program administration that have been identified as important or challenging to other organizations that have developed MST programs. These areas include, for example, quality control and evaluation, program financing, staff recruitment and retention, and youth referral and discharge criteria. In addition, programmatic features central to the success of MST programs (e.g., on-call systems, intraagency communication, interagency relations) are discussed, as are technological and practical needs (e.g., agency vehicles, insurance, cellular phones). Finally, appendices are provided that facilitate MST program development administratively. These include cost-estimating forms, job descriptions, recommendations for forming a community advisory board, and so forth.

## TRAINING

The core training package for formal MST programs is provided by MST Services, which has the exclusive license for the transport of MST technology and intellectual property through the Medical University of South Carolina. This package consists of pretraining organizational assessment and assistance, initial 5-day orientation training, weekly MST clinical consultation for each team of MST clinicians, and quarterly booster trainings. The training package was developed to replicate the characteristics of clinicians, training, clinical supervision, consultation, and program support provided in the successful clinical trials of MST with serious juvenile offenders. Chapters 5–7 described the adaptations in this package that are needed to serve youths with serious emotional disturbance.

## Pretraining and Assistance

Prior to MST training, consultation is provided regarding the development and implementation of a successful MST program. The objectives of this assessment are to identify the mission, policies, and practices of the provider organization and of the community context in which it operates; and to specify the clinical, organizational, fiscal, and community resources needed to successfully implement MST. Assessment activities include on-site meetings with the organization's leadership and clinical staff as well as meetings with staff from agencies that influence patterns of referral, reimbursement, and policy affecting the provider organization's capacity to implement MST. A central purpose of these meetings is to identify the goals of the MST program and outcomes for which the program will be accountable. In addition, assistance is provided in designing clinical record-keeping systems to document MST treatment goals and progress; reviewing evaluation proposals; measuring outcomes; and consulting on requests for proposals relevant to the development and funding of an MST program.

## Outcome Measurement

Significant effort is directed toward helping key stakeholders in each community identify ultimate outcomes for which the MST provider will be accountable. These outcomes are specified in a document entitled "MST Goals and Guidelines," which is generated during the pretraining site assessment. This document, which is "individualized" to each provider, specifies the domains in which outcomes are to be achieved, the criteria used to measure outcome attainment, the comparison against which outcomes will be measured, and the intervals of outcomes measurement (e.g., at baseline, posttreatment, at 6, 12, or 18 months posttreatment). Desired ultimate outcomes typically include reductions in out-of-home placements and costs, as well as improved individual, family, and school functioning. These outcomes reflect the domains proposed in a comprehensive model for treatment effectiveness described by Hoagwood and colleagues (Hoagwood, Jensen, Petti, & Burns, 1996) and are consistent with those endorsed by a broad constituency of policymakers, providers, consumers, and researchers (American College of Mental Health Administration, 1998).

Outcomes are often quantified in terms of benchmarks that represent significant change from previous years' rates of placement or in terms of rates achieved by alternative programs available in the community. Consultation on outcome measurement methods is provided during the site assessment process and as needed thereafter. Unfortunately, recent feedback from community-based MST providers indicated that many have no hard data on posttreatment outcomes. Barriers to data collection include insufficient resources (staff time); inadequate understanding of data collection procedures; and the satisfaction of families, referral sources (e.g., judges, agency directors, other staff) and payer agencies with the MST program, which mitigates against a sense of urgency to obtain hard data about outcomes. In response to this feedback from providers and referral agencies, the cost of administrative staff time required to obtain outcome data is now estimated for new providers and built into the quality assurance package. In addition, a semiannual review of new MST programs, which includes assessment of adherence and outcomes tracking mechanisms and prompts technical assistance with these tasks, is conducted.

## Initial 5-Day Training

Five days of initial orientation and training are provided for all clinical staff who will engage in treatment and/or clinical supervision of MST cases (e.g., psychiatrists, psychologists, therapists). This initial training includes didactic and experiential components. Didactic components include (1) instruction in systems theories, social learning theory, and the major psychological and sociological models and research regarding serious clinical problems in youth; (2) research relevant to problems experience by targeted youth (e.g., learning disabilities, depression, substance abuse); and (3) research on the evidence-based interventions used in MST. Experiential components include role plays on engagement, assessment, and intervention strategies and exercises designed to stimulate critical thinking about the treatment process (e.g., what evidence therapists use to draw conclusions about the correlates and causes of problems, how to determine whether interventions are effective). The overall intent of this 5-day training is to orient the participants to the MST model.

## Weekly Telephone Clinical Consultation

A core feature of the MST training program is the weekly telephone consultation with an MST expert (noted previously). One hour of phone time per week is dedicated to consultation for each team of three or four clinicians and their clinical supervisor. Teams fax weekly MST case summaries to consultants prior to the scheduled consultation time. The overarching objective of weekly telephone consultation is to facilitate therapist and supervisor adherence to MST. Whereas the provider organization's clinical supervisor and MST team are responsible for day-to-day decision making regarding case particulars, the MST consultant is responsible for contributing to the rapid and sustained development of the clinicians' ability to bring MST-like thinking and interventions to the cases. In so doing, the MST consultant identifies obstacles to implementing MST and suggests strategies to address these issues. When the obstacles appear related to the therapist, team, clinical supervisor, or consultant, recommendations can be made during the telephone consultation. When obstacles are related to organizational, community, fiscal, or policy issues, the consultant signals these possibilities to the appropriate audience (e.g., clinical supervisor, administrator, leadership of provider organization, state official contracting with provider) and assists the organization in developing strategies to overcome these obstacles.

## Quarterly Booster Training

As therapists gain field experience with MST, quarterly booster sessions are conducted on site. The purpose of these 1.5-day boosters is to provide additional training in areas identified by therapists and supervisors (e.g., marital interventions, treatment of caregiver depression) and to facilitate in-depth examination of, enactment, and problem solving concerning particularly difficult cases.

# CONTINUOUS QUALITY IMPROVEMENT SYSTEM

One of the long-term goals of the MST quality assurance system is to test and refine strategies that track treatment fidelity, youth outcomes, and the link between the two on a continuous basis. The validation of such an information system would allow consultants and program administrators to identify those therapists, supervisors, and teams that are achieving desired results as well as counterparts who are not. Additional training resources could then be selectively targeted at therapists and supervisors who are not attaining desired outcomes, while merit incentives can be used to reward those practitioners and supervisors who are successful. This section describes progress toward the development of an MST Continuous Quality Improvement (CQI) system.

## Therapist Adherence Measure

Therapist adherence to the nine principles of MST and the MST clinical process is assessed using the 26-item Likert-format MST Therapist Adherence Measure (TAM; see Table 9.1; Henggeler & Borduin, 1992). Ratings of therapist adherence are obtained from caregivers by phone 2 weeks after the start of treatment and once per month thereafter. For families without phones, supervisors or administrative staff at the provider agency conduct live interviews or have the caregiver return the TAM by mail. Data are entered into a database via an Internet-based system at *www.mstinstitute.org*. Adherence score reports are generated quarterly and discussed by the consultant, supervisor, and therapist at booster training sessions.

The TAM was originally developed by expert consensus. Analyses of data collected in two randomized trials showed that caregiver reports of high adherence on the TAM during treatment were associated with low rates of rearrest and incarceration of chronic juvenile offenders at a 1.7-year follow-up (Henggeler, Melton, et al., 1997) and with decreased criminal activity and out-of-home placement in substance-abusing juvenile offenders approximately 12 months postreferral (Henggeler, Pickrel, & Brondino, 1999). Using data from these two randomized trials, findings from Huey et al. (2000) and Schoenwald, Henggeler, Brondino, and Rowland (2000) supported the view that therapist adherence to MST principles influences those processes (e.g., family relations, association with deviant peers) that sustain adolescent antisocial behavior. Thus, empirical support for the association between therapist behavior and youth outcomes in clinical trials has been established.

## Supervisor Adherence Measure

Supervisor adherence to the MST supervisory protocol is assessed using the 43-item Likert-format MST Supervisor Adherence Measure (SAM; see Table 9.2; Schoenwald, Henggeler, & Edwards, 1998). The SAM was developed by expert consensus and is based on the rational constructs of supervision described in the MST Supervisory Manual (Henggeler & Schoenwald, 1998). Therapists provide ratings of their supervisors by completing the SAM at 2-month intervals, beginning 1 month after their first MST supervision session. Similar to the TAM, data from the SAM are entered into a database via an Internet-based system at

## TABLE 9.1. Therapist Adherence Measure

1. The session was lively and energetic.
2. The therapist tried to understand how my family's problems all fit together.
3. My family and the therapist worked together effectively.
4. My family knew exactly which problems we were working on.
5. The therapist recommended that family members do specific things to solve our problems.
6. The therapist's recommendations required family members to work on our problems almost every day.
7. My family and the therapist had similar ideas about ways to solve problems.
8. The therapist tried to change some ways that family members interact with each other.
9. The therapist tried to change some ways that family members interact with people outside the family.
10. My family and the therapist were honest and straightforward with each other.
11. The therapist's recommendations should help the children to mature.
12. Family members and the therapist agreed upon the goals of the session.
13. My family talked with the therapist about how well we followed his or her recommendations from the previous session.
14. My family talked with the therapist about the success (or lack of success) of his or her recommendations from the previous session.
15. The therapy session included a lot of irrelevant small talk (chit-chat).
16. We didn't get much accomplished during the therapy session.
17. Family members were engaged in power struggles with the therapist.
18. The therapist's recommendations required us to do almost all the work.
19. The therapy session was boring.
20. The family was not sure about the direction of treatment.
21. The therapist understood what is good about our family.
22. The therapist's recommendations made good use of our family's strengths.
23. My family accepted that part of the therapist's job is to help us change certain things about our family.
24. During the session, we talked about some experiences that occurred in previous sessions.
25. The therapist's recommendations should help family members to become more responsible.
26. There were awkward silences and pauses during the session.

## TABLE 9.2. Supervisor Adherence Measure

1. When the supervisor recommended changes in my course of action, the rationale for the recommendation was described in terms of one or more of the MST principles.
2. You could tell that the supervisor was in charge of the sessions.
3. Team members took a long time to describe the details of cases before the supervisor spoke.
4. The supervisor asked clinicians for evidence to support their hypotheses about the causes of problems targeted for change or of barriers to intervention success.
5. The supervisor asked clinicians how descriptions of this week's case developments pertained to identification of barriers to success.
6. When clinicians talked about events in the distant past, the supervisor recommended that current interactions within the family and between family members and others be examined first.
7. When clinicians reported on a variety of interventions tried during the week, the supervisor asked for clarification regarding which intermediary goals the interventions aimed to address.
8. The supervisor followed up on recommendations made in previous supervision sessions.
9. When interventions were not successful, discussion focused on identifying the barriers to success and actions the clinician should take to overcome them.
10. I have the skills to implement all of the recommendations made in supervision.
11. Interventions that were discussed targeted sequences of interaction between family members.
12. Clinicians received positive feedback during the sessions.
13. When interventions were not successful, the supervisor asked clinicians to describe the details of the intervention and steps clinicians took to assure implementation and monitoring of results.
14. The supervisor asked clinicians how descriptions and questions about case developments pertained to fit assessment.
15. It was easy for team members to acknowledge frustrations, mistakes, and failures.
16. When a clinician presented information about events that transpired during the week, the supervisor asked the clinician and team to clarify the relevance of the information to one or more steps of the analytical process.
17. Weekly case summaries were referred to during the discussion of cases.
18. Interventions that were discussed targeted sequences of interaction between family members and individuals at school, in the child's peer group, or in the neighborhood.
19. When an intervention was only partially successful, the supervisor asked questions to determine whether the clinician had adequately and completely implemented the intervention.
20. We spent more time discussing cases in which progress was limited.
21. When an intervention was only partially successful, the supervisor asked questions to determine whether the clinician had provided participants with the understanding, skills, and practice needed to implement the intervention.

*(continued)*

**TABLE 9.2.** (*continued*)

22. The supervisor referred to specific MST principles while discussing cases.

23. The supervisor made a note of case-specific recommendations.

24. When new areas were targeted for intervention, the supervisor encouraged the clinician to articulate new intermediary goals accordingly.

25. Outcomes were described in observable and measurable terms.

26. When clinicians reported plans to meet with teachers, neighbors, or officials from other agencies, the supervisor asked what it would take for a caregiver to hold the meeting.

27. When clinicians reported that things were going well in a case, the supervisor focused discussion on factors in the natural ecology that were sustaining progress.

28. When clinicians reported doing things for family members, the supervisor asked what it would take for family members to do these things for themselves.

29. When clinicians reported that they discussed a particular problem with a family, the supervisor asked what plans were put in place to address the problem this week.

30. When clinicians described their ideas about the causes of problems, "fit circles" were developed and discussed in session.

31. When clinicians talked about events in the distant past, the supervisor asked for evidence that these events are contributing to a current problem.

32. The supervisor had difficulty managing team discussion.

33. In the past 2 months, the supervisor and I have discussed the extent to which my case summaries and in-session presentations are consistent with the MST principles and analytic process.

34. In the past 2 months, the supervisor and I have set goals for development of my specific competencies in MST.

35. In the past 2 months, my supervisor has accompanied me to therapy sessions (i.e., field supervision) *or* reviewed audiotapes of my therapy sessions.

36. In the past 2 months, the supervisor and I have discussed my strengths and needs with respect to adherence to the 9 MST principles.

37. In the past 2 months, I left supervision knowing how to carry out recommended actions.

38. How knowledgeable do you think your supervisor is in the theory of MST?

39. How skilled do you think your supervisor is in treatment modalities used in MST such as behavior therapy?

40. How skilled do you think your supervisor is in implementing MST interventions?

41. How skilled do you think your supervisor is in the treatment modalities used in MST such as cognitive-behavioral therapy?

42. How often does team (group) supervision occur?

43. How often have you and your supervisor met to develop and monitor a plan to help you increase your knowledge and skill in MST?

*www.mstinstitute.org*. Evidence supporting the association between therapist and supervisor adherence is emerging from multisite studies of MST programs (Henggeler, Schoenwald, Liao, Letourneau, & Edwards, 2002; Schoenwald, 2000).

## Investigating Additional Linkages in the Quality Assurance System

As noted above, two of the key associations in the MST quality assurance system (i.e., the therapist–family linkage, the supervisor–therapist linkage) have been supported empirically. The influence of other aspects of the MST quality assurance system remains to be determined, however. Key examples include the hypothesized association between consultant behavior and the functioning of MST teams as well as the impact of organizational characteristics on the ability of therapists and supervisors to follow MST treatment guidelines. Research currently underway will help answer these questions. One project, funded by the NIMH (Schoenwald, principal investigator) is examining the relationship of therapist adherence to child outcomes in 41 community-based MST programs and the impact of therapist, supervisory, organizational, and interagency factors on therapist fidelity to MST. Data regarding consultation provided to these programs are being collected, such that potential links between consultation, supervision, and therapist adherence can be examined for the first time.

## INTERNAL CAPACITY BUILDING

A major goal of the research efforts described above is to determine what is needed to develop the internal capacity of a service system to implement successful MST programs on a relatively large scale. At issue here is how systems can develop the expertise needed to move from a discrete MST program in one community to a scenario in which all counties in a state or province that needed an MST program would have one. MST Services, the university-affiliated organization established to facilitate the quality-controlled dissemination of MST, is at the forefront of these efforts. One model of capacity building currently being implemented in Norway involves three phases. In the first phase, a new MST program is established in a community, and MST Services provides all the training, consultation, and quality assurance procedures described earlier. In the second phase, additional therapists are hired (thus adding capacity to serve more youths), and performance and outcome criteria are used to promote the most successful therapists from the original teams to supervisory positions, and the most successful supervisors to internal MST consultant status. During this second phase, MST Services provides training and consultation to newly promoted internal system consultants, who provide consultation to newly hired therapists and supervisors. During the third phase, the internal consultants provide training and support to supervisors and therapists, with technical assistance provided by MST Services only as indicated on the basis of problematic adherence and outcome data or upon request. By tracking the adherence and outcomes achieved at each phase, it should be possible to detect whether the transfer of expertise needed to sustain successful MST programs is occurring.

Similar approaches are being developed in Canada, Ohio, Connecticut, Colorado, and South Carolina. In Ohio, for example, key stakeholders in the state and county mental health system are developing a state-sponsored center for training and implementation of evidence-based mental health practices throughout the state. MST is a centerpiece for this endeavor, and the phasic model of capacity building described for Norway is also being considered as part of those plans. Regardless of the particular model pursued, helping communities to develop the internal capacity needed to implement effective treatments for youth with serious emotional disturbances and their families is a priority; and a combination of dissemination, quality assurance, and research efforts are being directed toward that goal by investigators at the Medical University of South Carolina and other leading universities.

## CONCLUSION

Although quality improvement systems have proven invaluable in many segments of the nation's economy, such systems are extremely rare in the mental health arena. Yet logic and our own experience suggest that quality assurance (and improvement) systems hold great promise in the promotion of improved clinical outcomes for youths with serious emotional disturbance and their families. Similarly, such systems can provide funders and policymakers with a level accountability that is desired, but currently lacking.

# References

American Academy of Child and Adolescent Psychiatry. (1997). Practice standards for the assessment and treatment of children and adolescents with bipolar disorder. *Journal of the American Academy of Child and Adolescent Psychiatry, 36*(Suppl.), 157S–176S.

American Academy of Child and Adolescent Psychiatry. (1998). Practice standards for the assessment and treatment of children and adolescents with posttraumatic stress disorder. *Journal of the American Academy of Child and Adolescent Psychiatry, 37*(Suppl.), 4S–26S.

American College of Mental Health Administration. (1998). *Preserving quality and value in the managed care equation.* Pittsburgh: Author.

American Psychiatric Association. (1994). *Diagnostic and statistical manual of mental disorders* (4th ed.). Washington, DC: Author.

Anhalt, K., McNeil, C. B., & Bahl, A. B. (1998). The ADHD Classroom Kit: A whole-classroom approach for managing disruptive behavior. *Psychology in the Schools, 35,* 67–79.

Aos, S., Phipps, P., Barnoski, R., & Lieb, R. (1999). *The comparative costs and benefits of programs to reduce crime: A review of national research findings with implications for Washington State, Version 3.0.* Olympia: Washington State Institute for Public Policy.

Apolloni, A. H., & Triest, G. (1983). Respite services in California: Status and recommendations for improvement. *Mental Retardation, 21,* 240–243.

Armsden, G. C., & Greenberg, M. T. (1987). The Inventory of Parent and Peer Attachment: Individual differences and their relationship to psychological well-being in adolescence. *Journal of Youth and Adolescence, 16,* 427–454.

Armsden, G. C., McCauley, E., Greenberg, M. T., Burke, P. M., & Mitchell, J. R. (1990). Parent and peer attachment in early adolescent depression. *Journal of Abnormal Child Psychology, 18,* 683–697.

Arnold, M. E., & Hughes, J. N. (1999). First do no harm: Adverse effects of grouping deviant youth for skills training. *Journal of School Psychology, 37,* 99–115.

Ary, D. V., Duncan, T. E., Duncan, S. C., & Hops, H. (1999). Adolescent problem behavior: The influence of parents and peers. *Behaviour Research and Therapy, 37,* 217–230.

Asarnow, J. R., & Asarnow, R. F. (1996). Childhood-onset schizophrenia. In E. J. Mash & R. A. Barkley (Eds.), *Child psychopathology* (pp. 340–361). New York: Guilford Press.

Athanasou, J. (1994). Job finding in Australia. *Australian Journal of Career Development, 3,* 51–54.

Backer, T. E., & David, S. L. (1995). Synthesis of behavioral science learnings about technology transfer. *National Institute on Drug Abuse Monograph Series, 155* (pp. 262–279). Rockville, MD: U.S. Department of Health and Human Services.

Baker, B. L. (1983). Parents as teachers: Issues in training. In J. A. Mulnick & S. M. Pueschel (Eds.), *Parent–professional partnerships in development disability services* (pp. 55–74). Cambridge, MA: Ware Press.

Barker, P. (1998). The future of residential treatment for children. In C. Schaefer & A. Swanson (Eds.), *Children in residential care: Critical issues in treatment* (pp. 1–16). New York: Van Nostrand Reinhold.

Barkley, R. A. (1997). *Defiant children: A clinician's manual for assessment and parent training* (2nd ed.). New York: Guilford Press.

Barkley, R. A. (1998). *Attention-deficit hyperactivity disorder: A handbook for diagnosis and treatment* (2nd ed.). New York: Guilford Press.

Barkley, R. A. (2000). *Taking charge of ADHD: The complete, authoritative guide for parents* (rev. ed.), New York: Guilford Press.

Barrera, M., & Garrison-Jones, C. (1992). Family and peer support as specific correlates of adolescent depressive symptoms. *Journal of Abnormal Child Psychology, 20,* 1–16.

Barrett, P. M., Dadds, M. R., & Rapee, R. M. (1996). Family treatment of childhood anxiety: A controlled trial. *Journal of Consulting and Clinical Psychology, 64,* 333–342.

Baumrind, D. (1989). Rearing competent children. In W. Damon (Ed.), *Child development today and tomorrow* (pp. 349–378). San Francisco, CA: Jossey-Bass.

Beck, J. S. (1995). *Cognitive therapy: Basics and beyond.* New York: Guilford Press.

Becker, J. V., Alpert, J. L., Bigfoot, D. S., Bonner, B. L., Geddie, L. F., Henggeler, S. W., Kaufman, K. L., & Walker, C. E. (1995). Empirical research on child abuse treatment: Report by the Child Abuse and Neglect Treatment Working Group, American Psychological Association. *Journal of Clinical Child Psychology, 24*(Suppl.), 23–46.

Belenko, S. (1998). Research on drug courts: A critical review. *National Drug Court Institute Review, 1,* 1–43.

Berman, A. L., & Jobes, D. A. (1992). Suicidal behavior of adolescents. In B. Bongar (Ed.), *Suicide: Guidelines for assessment, management, and treatment* (pp. 84–105). New York: Oxford University Press.

Bickman, L. (1999). Practice makes perfect and other myths about mental health services. *American Psychologist, 54,* 965–978.

Bickman, L., Noser, K., & Summerfelt, W. T. (1999). Long-term effects of a system of care on children and adolescents. *Journal of Behavioral Health Services and Research, 26,* 185–202.

Bickman, L., Summerfelt, W. T., & Noser, K. (1997). Comparative outcomes of emotionally disturbed children and adolescents in a system of services and usual care. *Psychiatric Services, 48,* 1543–1548.

Bierman, K. L., & Montminy, H. P. (1993). Developmental issues in social skills assessment and intervention with children and adolescents. *Behavior Modification, 17,* 229–254.

Birmaher, B., Ryan, N. D., Williamson, D. E., Brent, D. A., & Kaufman, J. (1996). Childhood and adolescent depression: A review of the past 10 years, Part II. *Journal of the American Academy of Child and Adolescent Psychiatry, 35,* 1575–1583.

Birmaher, B., Ryan, N. D., Williamson, D. E., Brent, D. A., Kaufman, J., Dahl, R. E., Perel, J., & Nelson, B. (1996). Childhood and adolescent depression: A review of the past 10 years, Part I. *Journal of the American Academy of Child and Adolescent Psychiatry, 35,* 1427–1439.

Boothroyd, R. A., Kuppinger, A. D., Evans, M. E., Armstrong, M. I., & Radigan, M. (1998). Understanding respite care use by families of children receiving short-term in-home psychiatric emergency services. *Journal of Child and Family Studies, 7,* 353–376.

Borduin, C. M., Henggeler, S. W., Blaske, D. M., & Stein, R. (1990). Multisystemic treatment of adolescent sexual offenders. *International Journal of Offender Therapy and Comparative Criminology, 35,* 105–114.

Borduin, C. M., Mann, B. J., Cone, L. T., Henggeler, S. W., Fucci, B. R., Blaske, D. M., & Williams, R. A. (1995). Multisystemic treatment of serious juvenile offenders: Long-term prevention of criminality and violence. *Journal of Consulting and Clinical Psychology, 63,* 569–578.

Borduin, C. M., Schaeffer, C. M., & Heiblum, N. (2002). *Multisystemic treatment of aggressive and nonaggressive sexual offending in adolescents: Instrumental and ultimate outcomes.* Manuscript in preparation.

Boyd, J. H., & Moscicki, E. K. (1986). Firearms and youth suicide. *American Journal of Public Health, 76,* 1240–1242.

Brent, D. A., Kolko, D. J., Allan, M. J., & Brown, R. V. (1990). Suicidality in affectively disordered adolescent inpatients. *Journal of the American Academy of Child and Adolescent Psychiatry, 29,* 586–593.

Brent, D. A., Kolko, D. J., Wartella, M. E., Boylan, M. B., Moritz, G., Baugher, M., & Zelenak, J. P. (1993). Adolescent psychiatric inpatients' risk of suicide attempt at 6–month follow-up. *Journal of the American Academy of Child and Adolescent Psychiatry, 32,* 95–105.

Brent, D. A., Perper, J. A., & Allman, C. (1987). Alcohol, firearms and suicide among youth: Temporal trends in Allegheny County, Pennsylvania, 1960 to 1983. *Journal of the American Medical Association, 257,* 3369–3372.

Brent, D. A., Perper, J. A., Goldstein, C. E., Kolko, D. J., Allan, M. J., Allman, C. J., & Zelenak, J. P. (1988). Risk factors for adolescent suicide. *Archives of General Psychiatry, 45,* 581–588.

Bronfenbrenner, U. (1979). *The ecology of human development: Experiments by design and nature.* Cambridge, MA: Harvard University Press.

Brown, B. S. (1995). Reducing impediments to technology transfer in drug abuse programming. *National Institute on Drug Abuse Monograph Series, 155* (pp. 169–185). Rockville, MD: U.S. Department of Health and Human Services.

Brown, T. L., Henggeler, S. W., Schoenwald, S. K., Brondino, M. J., & Pickrel, S. G. (1999). Multisystemic treatment of substance abusing and dependent juvenile delinquents: Effects on school attendance at posttreatment and 6–month follow-up. *Children's Services: Social Policy, Research, and Practice, 2,* 81–93.

Brunk, M., Henggeler, S. W., & Whelan, J. P. (1987). A comparison of multisystemic therapy and parent training in the brief treatment of child abuse and neglect. *Journal of Consulting and Clinical Psychology, 55,* 311–318.

Budney, A. J., & Higgins, S. T. (1998). *A community reinforcement plus vouchers approach: Treating cocaine addiction* (Pub. No. NIH 98–4309). Washington, DC: National Institutes of Health, U.S. Department of Health and Human Services.

Burns, B. J. (1991). Mental health service use by adolescents in the 1970s and 1980s. *Journal of the American Academy of Child and Adolescent Psychiatry, 30,* 144–150.

Burns, B. J., Compton, S. N., Egger, H. L., & Farmer, E. M. (2000). *An annotated review of the evidence base for psychosocial and psychopharmacological interventions for children with attention-deficit/hyperactivity disorder, major depressive disorder, disruptive behavior disorders, anxiety disorders, and posttraumatic stress disorder.* Durham, NC: Department of Psychiatry and Behavioral Sciences, Duke University Medical Center.

Burns, B. J., Hoagwood, K., & Mrazek, P. J. (1999). Effective treatment for mental disorders in children and adolescents. *Clinical Child and Family Psychology Review, 2,* 199–254.

Campbell, M., Gonzalez, N. M., Ernst, M., Silva, R. R., & Werry, J. S. (1993). Antipsychotics (neuroleptics). In J. S. Werry & M. G. Aman (Eds.), *Practitioner's guide to psychoactive drugs for children and adolescents* (pp. 269–296). New York: Plenum Medical Press.

Center for Substance Abuse Prevention (CSAP). (2000). *Strengthening America's families: Model family programs for substance abuse and delinquency prevention.* Salt Lake City: Department of Health Promotion and Education, University of Utah.

Chase-Lansdale, P. L., Brooks-Gunn, J., & Zamsky, E. S. (1994). Young African-American multigenerational families in poverty: Quality of mothering and grandmothering. *Child Development, 65,* 373–393.

Cicchetti, D. L., & Toth, S. L. (1995). Developmental psychopathology and disorders of affect. In D. L. Cicchetti & D. J. Cohen (Eds.), *Developmental psychopathology: Risk, disorder, and adaptation* (Vol. 2, pp. 369–420). New York: Wiley.

Cohen, S. (1982). Supporting families through respite care. *Rehabilitation Literature, 43,* 7–11.

Cohen-Sandler, R., Berman, A. L., & King, R. A. (1982). Life stress and symptomatology: Determinants of suicidal behavior in children. *Journal of the American Academy of Child Psychiatry, 21,* 178–186.

Conners, C. K., Sitarenios, G., Parker, J. D. A., & Epstein, J. N. (1998). Revision and restandardization of the Conners Teacher Rating Scale (CTRS-R): Factor structure, reliability, and criterion validity. *Journal of Abnormal Child Psychology, 26,* 279–291.

Crook, T., Raskin, A., & Eliot, J. (1981). Parent–child relationships and adult depression. *Child Development, 52,* 950–957.

Cummings, E. M., & Davies, P. T. (1994). *Children and marital conflict: The impact of family dispute and resolution.* New York: Guilford Press.

Cunningham, P. B., & Henggeler, S. W. (1999). Engaging multiproblem families in treatment: Lessons learned throughout the development of multisystemic therapy. *Family Process, 38,* 265–281.

Cunningham, P. B., & Henggeler, S. W. (2001). Implementation of an empirically-based drug and violence prevention and intervention program in public school settings. *Journal of Clinical Child Psychology, 30,* 221–232.

Davis, J. M., Comaty, J. E., & Janicak, P. G. (1987). The psychological effects of antipsychotic drugs. In C. N. Stefanis & A. D. Rabavilas (Eds.), *Schizophrenia: Recent biosocial developments* (pp. 165–181). New York: Human Sciences Press.

Day, C., & Roberts, M. C. (1991). Activities of the Children and Adolescent Services System Program for improving mental health services for children and families. *Journal of Clinical Child Psychology, 20,* 340–350.

Dishion, T. J., McCord, J., & Poulin, F. (1999). When interventions harm: Peer groups and problem behavior. *American Psychologist, 54,* 755–764.

Dunn, L. M., & Markwardt, F. C., Jr. (1970). *Peabody Individual Achievement Test.* Circle Pines, MN: American Guidance Services.

Dunn, R. L., & Schwebel, A. I. (1995). Meta-analytic review of marital therapy outcome research. *Journal of Family Psychology, 9,* 58–68.

Elliott, D. S. (Series Ed.). (1998). *Blueprints for violence prevention.* Boulder, CO: Blueprints Publications.

Elliott, D. S., Huizinga, D., & Ageton, S. S. (1985). *Explaining delinquency and drug use.* Beverly Hills, CA: Sage.

Ellis, D. A., Naar-King, S., Frey, M., Greger, N., & Arfken, C. (2000). *Therapy in IDDM adolescents in poor metabolic control.* Detroit, MI: Children's Hospital of Michigan, Wayne State University.

Emery, R. E. (1994). *Renegotiating family relationships: Divorce, child custody, and mediation.* New York: Guilford Press.

Emery, R. E. (1999). *Marriage, divorce, and children's adjustment* (2nd ed.). Thousand Oaks, CA: Sage.

Emslie, G. J., Walkup, J. T., Pliszka, S. R., & Ernst, M. (1999). Nontricyclic antidepressants: Current trends in children and adolescents. *Journal of the American Academy of Child and Adolescent Psychiatry, 38,* 517–528.

Erickson, D. H., Beiser, M., Iacono, W. G., Fleming, J. A., & Lin, T. (1989). The role of social relationships in the course of first-episode schizophrenia and affective psychosis. *American Journal of Psychiatry, 146,* 1456–1461.

Evans, M. E., Armstrong, M. I., & Kuppinger, A. D. (1996). Family-centered intensive case management: A step toward understanding individualized care. *Journal of Child and Family Studies, 5,* 55–65.

Fagan, J., & Wexler, S. (1987). Family origins of violent delinquents. *Criminology, 25,* 643–669.

Farmer, T. W., Farmer, E. M. Z., & Gut, D. M. (1999). Implications of social development research for school-based interventions for aggressive youth with EBD. *Journal of Emotional and Behavioral Disorders, 7,* 130–137.

Farrington, D. P., & Welsh, B. C. (1999). Delinquency prevention using family-based interventions. *Children and Society, 13,* 287–303.

Fine, M. J., & Carlson, C. (Eds.) (1992). *The handbook of family–school intervention: A systems perspective.* Needham Heights, MA: Allyn & Bacon.

Foa, E. B., Keane, E. M., & Friedman, M. J. (Eds.). (2000). *Effective treatments for PTSD: Practice guidelines from the International Society for Traumatic Stress Studies.* New York: Guilford Press.

Foster, S. L., & Robin, A. L. (1998). Parent–adolescent conflict and relationship discord. In E. J. Mash & R. A. Barkley (Eds.), *Treatment of childhood disorders* (2nd ed., pp. 601–646). New York: Guilford Press.

Fraser, M. W., Nelson, K. E., & Rivard, J. C. (1997). Effectiveness of family preservation services. *Social Work Research, 2,* 138–153.

Gendreau, P. (1996). Offender rehabilitation: What we know and what needs to be done. *Criminal Justice and Behavior, 23,* 144–161.

Gendreau, P., & Goggin, C. (1997). Correctional treatment: Accomplishments and realities. In P. Van Voorhis, M. Braswell, & D. Lester (Eds.), *Correctional counseling and rehabilitation* (3rd ed., pp. 271–279). Cincinnati: Anderson.

Gispert, M., Davis, M. S., Marsh, L., & Wheeler, K. (1987). Predictive factors in repeated suicide attempts by adolescents. *Hospital and Community Psychiatry, 38,* 390–393.

Glisson, C., & Hemmelgarn, A. L. (1998). The effects of organizational climate and interorganizational coordination on the quality and outcomes of children's service systems. *Child Abuse and Neglect, 22,* 401–421.

Gotlib, I. H., Lewinsohn, P. M., Seeley, J. R., Rohde, P., & Redner, J. E. (1993). Negative cognitions and attributional style in depressed adolescents: An examination of stability and specificity. *Journal of Abnormal Psychology, 102,* 607–615.

Gottfredson, S. D., & Gottfredson, D. M. (1988). Violence prediction methods: Statistical and clinical strategies. *Violence and Victims, 3,* 303–324.

Graham, P., & Rutter, M. (1985). Adolescent disorders. In M. Rutter & K. Hersov (Eds.), *Child and adolescent psychiatry: Modern approaches.* Oxford, UK: Blackwell Scientific Publications.

Green, W. H. (1995). *Child and adolescent psychopharmacology* (2nd ed.). Baltimore: Williams & Wilkins.

Greenhill, L. L., Abikoff, H. B., Arnold, L. E., Cantwell, D. P., Conners, C. K., Elliott, G., Hechtman, L., Hinshaw, S. P., Hoza, B., Jensen, P. S., March, J. S., Newcorn, J., Pelham, W. E., Severe, J. B., Swanson, J. M., Vitiello, B., & Wells, K. (1996). Medication treatment strategies in the MTA study: Relevance to clinicians and researchers. *Journal of the American Academy of Child and Adolescent Psychiatry, 34,* 1304–1313.

Haley, J. (1976). *Problem solving therapy.* San Francisco: Jossey-Bass.

Halliday-Boykins, C. A., & Henggeler, S. W. (2001). Multisystemic therapy: Theory, Research, and Practice. In E. Walton, P. A. Sandau-Beckler, & M. Mannes (Eds.), *Balancing family-centered services and child well-being* (pp. 320–335). New York: Columbia University Press.

Halpern, P. L. (1985). Respite care and family functioning in families with retarded children. *Health and Social Work, 10,* 138–150.

Hawkins, J. D., Catalano, R. F., & Miller, J. Y. (1992). Risk and protective factors for alcohol and other drug problems in adolescence and early adulthood: Implications for substance abuse prevention. *Psychological Bulletin, 112,* 64–105.

Hawton, K., Osborn, M., O'Grady, J., & Cole, D. (1982). Classification of adolescents who take overdoses. *British Journal of Psychiatry, 140,* 124–131.

Henegan, A. M., Horwitz, S. M., & Leventhal, J. M. (1997). Evaluation of intensive family preservation programs: A methodological review. *Pediatrics, 97,* 535–542.

Henggeler, S. W. (1997a). *Juvenile justice bulletin—Treating serious antisocial behavior in youth: The MST approach.* Washington, DC: Office of Juvenile Justice and Delinquency Prevention, U.S. Department of Justice.

Henggeler, S. W. (1997b). The development of effective drug abuse services for youth. In J. A. Egertson, D. M. Fox, & A. I. Leshner (Eds.), *Treating drug abusers effectively* (pp. 253–279). New York: Blackwell North America/Milbank Memorial Fund.

Henggeler, S. W., & Borduin, C. M. (1992). *Multisystemic Therapy Adherence Scales.* Unpublished instrument, Department of Psychiatry and Behavioral Sciences, Medical University of South Carolina.

Henggeler, S. W., & Borduin, C. M., Melton, G. B., Mann, B. J., Smith, L., Hall, J. A., Cone, L., & Fucci, B. R. (1991). Effects of multisystemic therapy on drug use and abuse in serious juvenile offenders: A progress report from two outcome studies. *Family Dynamics of Addiction Quarterly, 1,* 40–51.

Henggeler, S. W., Clingempeel, W. G., Brondino, M. J., & Pickrel, S. G. (in press). Four-year follow-up of multisystemic therapy with substance abusing and dependent juvenile offenders. *Journal of the American Academy of Child and Adolescent Psychiatry.*

Henggeler, S. W., Melton, G. B., Brondino, M. J., Scherer, D. G., & Hanley, J. H. (1997). Multisystemic therapy with violent and chronic juvenile offenders and their families: The role of treatment fidelity in successful dissemination. *Journal of Consulting and Clinical Psychology, 65,* 821–833.

Henggeler, S. W., Melton, G. B., & Smith, L. A. (1992). Family preservation using multisystemic therapy: An effective alternative to incarcerating serious juvenile offenders. *Journal of Consulting and Clinical Psychology, 60,* 953–961.

Henggeler, S. W., Melton, G. B., Smith, L. A., Schoenwald, S. K., & Hanley, J. H. (1993). Family preservation using multisystemic treatment: Long-term follow-up to a clinical trial with serious juvenile offenders. *Journal of Child and Family Studies, 2,* 283–293.

Henggeler, S. W., Pickrel, S. G., & Brondino, M. J. (1999). Multisystemic treatment of substance abusing and dependent delinquents: Outcomes, treatment fidelity, and transportability. *Mental Health Services Research, 1,* 171–184.

Henggeler, S. W., Pickrel, S. G., Brondino, M. J., & Crouch, J. L. (1996). Eliminating (almost) treatment dropout of substance abusing or dependent delinquents through home-based multisystemic therapy. *American Journal of Psychiatry, 153,* 427–428.

Henggeler, S. W., Rodick, J. D., Borduin, C. M., Hanson, C. L., Watson, S. M., & Urey, J. R. (1986). Multisystemic treatment of juvenile offenders: Effects on adolescent behavior and family interactions. *Developmental Psychology, 22,* 132–141.

Henggeler, S. W., Rowland, M. D., Pickrel, S. G., Miller, S. L., Cunningham, P. B., Santos, A. B., Schoenwald, S. K., Randall, J., & Edwards, J. E. (1997). Investigating family-based alternatives to institution-based mental health services for youth: Lessons learned from the pilot study of a randomized field trial. *Journal of Clinical Child Psychology, 26,* 226–233.

Henggeler, S. W., Rowland, M. R., Randall, J., Ward, D., Pickrel, S. G., Cunningham, P. B., Miller, S. L., Edwards, J. E., Zealberg, J., Hand, L., & Santos, A. B. (1999). Home-based multisystemic therapy as an alternative to the hospitalization of youth in psychiatric crisis: Clinical outcomes. *Journal of the American Academy of Child and Adolescent Psychiatry, 38,* 1331–1339.

Henggeler, S. W., & Schoenwald, S. K. (1998). *The MST supervisory manual: Promoting quality assurance at the clinical level.* Charleston, SC: MST Services, Inc.

Henggeler, S. W., & Schoenwald, S. K. (1999). The role of quality assurance in achieving outcomes in MST programs. *Journal of Juvenile Justice and Detention Services, 14,* 1–17.

Henggeler, S. W., Schoenwald, S. K., Borduin, C. M., Rowland, M. D., & Cunningham, P. B. (1998). *Multisystemic treatment of antisocial behavior in children and adolescents.* New York: Guilford Press.

Henggeler, S. W., Schoenwald, S. K., Liao, J. G., Letourneau, E. J., & Edwards, D. L. (2002). Transporting efficacious treatments to field settings: The link between supervisory practices and therapist fidelity in MST programs. *Journal of Clinical Child Psychology, 31,* 155–167.

Henggeler, S. W., Schoenwald, S. K., & Munger, R. L. (1996). Families and therapists achieve outcomes, systems of care mediate the process. *Journal of Child and Family Studies, 5,* 177–183.

Hetherington, E. M., & Clingempeel, W. G. (1992). Coping with marital transitions. *Monographs of the Society for Research in Child Development, 57,* 1–229.

Higgins, S. T., & Budney, A. J. (1993). Treatment of cocaine dependence through the principles of behavior analysis and behavioral pharmacology. In L. S. Onken, J. D. Blaine, & J. Boren, *Behavioral treatments for drug abuse and dependence*

*(National Institute on Drug Abuse Research Monograph 137*, NIH Publication No. 93–3684). Rockville, MD: National Institutes of Health.

Hoagwood, K. (2000). State of the evidence on school-based mental health services— NIMH perspectives. *Emotional and Behavioral Disorders in Youth, 1*(Winter), 13–15.

Hoagwood, K., Jensen, P. S., Petti, T., & Burns, B. J. (1996). Outcomes of mental health care for children and adolescents: A comprehensive conceptual model. *Journal of the American Academy of Child and Adolescent Psychiatry, 35,* 1055–1063.

Holden, G. W., & Miller, P. C. (1999). Enduring and different: A meta-analysis of the similarity in parents' child rearing. *Psychological Bulletin, 125,* 223–254.

Hops, H., Lewinsohn, P. M., Andrews, J. A., & Roberts, R. E. (1990). Psychosocial correlates of depressive symptomatology among high school students. *Journal of Clinical Child Psychology, 3,* 211–220.

House, J. S., Landis, K. R., & Umberson, D. (1988). Social relationships and health. *Science, 241,* 540–545.

Huey, S. J., Henggeler, S. W., Brondino, M. J., & Pickrel, S. G. (2000). Mechanisms of change in multisystemic therapy: Reducing delinquent behavior through therapist adherence and improved family and peer functioning. *Journal of Consulting and Clinical Psychology, 68,* 451–467.

Hughes, C. W., Emslie, G. J., Crismon, M. L., Wagner, K. D., Birmaher, B., Geller, B., Pliszka, S. R., Ryan, N. D., Strober, M., Trivedi, M. H., Toprac, M. G., Sedillo, A., Llana, M. E., Lopez, M., & Rush, A. J. (1999). The Texas Children's Medication Algorithm Project: Report of the Texas Consensus Conference Panel on Medication Treatment of Childhood Major Depressive Disorder. *Journal of the American Academy of Child and Adolescent Psychiatry, 38,* 1442–1454.

Jacobs, D. (1983). Evaluation and management of the violent patient in emergency settings. *Psychiatric Clinics of North America, 6,* 259–269.

Jastak, S., & Wilkinson, G. S. (1984). *Wide Range Achievement Test—Revised.* Wilmington, DE: Jastak.

Jensen, P. S. (Guest Ed.). (2001). Introduction: ADHD comorbidity and treatment outcomes in the MTA. *Journal of the American Academy of Child and Adolescent Psychiatry, 40,* 134–205. (Special section on the MTA.)

Joshi, P. K., & Rosenberg, L. A. (1997). Children's behavioral response to residential treatment. *Journal of Clinical Psychology, 53,* 567–573.

Joshi, P. T., Hamel, L., Joshi, A. R., & Capozzoli, J. A. (1998). Use of droperidol in hospitalized children. *Journal of the American Academy of Child and Adolescent Psychiatry, 37,* 228–230.

Joyce, K., & Singer, M. I. (1983). Respite care services: An evaluation of the perceptions of parents and workers. *Rehabilitation Literature, 44,* 270–274.

Kashani, J. H., Burbach, D. J., & Rosenberg, T. K. (1988). Perception of family conflict resolution and depressive symptomatology in adolescents. *Journal of the American Academy of Child and Adolescent Psychiatry, 27,* 42–48.

Kaslow, N. J., Deering, C. G., & Racusin, G. R. (1994). Depressed children and their families. *Clinical Psychology Review, 14,* 39–59.

Kazdin, A. E. (1982). *Single-case research designs: Methods for clinical and applied settings.* New York: Oxford University Press.

Kazdin, A. E. (1983). Psychiatric diagnosis, dimensions of dysfunction and child behavior therapy. *Behavior Therapy, 14,* 279–286.

Kazdin, A. E. (1990). Childhood depression. *Journal of Child Psychology and Psychiatry and Allied Disciplines, 31,* 121–160.

Kazdin, A. E. (1996). Problem solving and parent management in treating aggressive and antisocial behavior. In E. D. Hibbs & P. S. Jensen (Eds.), *Psychosocial treatments for child and adolescent disorders: Empirically based strategies for clinical practice* (pp. 377–408). Washington, DC: American Psychological Association.

Kazdin, A. E., Siegel, T. C., & Bass, D. (1992). Cognitive problem solving skills therapy and parent management training in the treatment of antisocial behavior in children. *Journal of Consulting and Clinical Psychology, 60,* 733–747.

Kazdin, A. E., & Weisz, J. R. (1998). Identifying and developing empirically supported child and adolescent treatments. *Journal of Consulting and Clinical Psychology, 66,* 19–36.

Kellermann, A. L., & Reay, D. T. (1986). Protection or peril? An analysis of firearm-related deaths in the home. *New England Journal of Medicine, 314,* 1557–1560.

Kendall, P. C., Flannery-Schroeder, E., Panichelli-Mindel, S. M., Southam-Gerow, M., Henin, A., & Warman, M. (1997). Therapy for youths with anxiety disorders: A second randomized clinical trial. *Journal of Consulting and Clinical Psychology, 65,* 366–380.

Kotila, L., & Lonnquist, J. (1989). Suicide and violent death among adolescent suicide attempters. *Acta Psychiatrica Scandinavica, 79,* 453–459.

Kovacs, M. (1992). *Children's Depression Inventory CDI manual.* Ontario: MHS Multi-Health Systems.

Leff, J. P., Kuipers, L., Berkowitz, R., & Sturgeon, D. (1985). A controlled trial of social intervention in the families of schizophrenic patients: Two year follow-up. *British Journal of Psychiatry, 146,* 594–600.

Leff, J., & Vaughn, C. (1981). The role of maintenance therapy and relatives' expressed emotion in relapse of schizophrenia: A two-year follow-up. *British Journal of Psychiatry, 139,* 102–104.

Lefkowitz, M. M., & Tesiny, E. P. (1984). Rejection and depression: Prospective and contemporaneous analyses. *Developmental Psychology, 20,* 776–785.

Leschied, A. W., & Cunningham, A. (2001). Intensive community-based services can influence re-offending rates of high-risk youth: Preliminary results of the multisystemic therapy clinical trials in Ontario. *Empirical and Applied Criminal Justice Research, 1,* 1–24.

Lester, D., & Murrell, M. E. (1980). The influence of gun control laws on suicidal behavior. *American Journal of Psychiatry, 137,* 121–122.

Liddle, H. A. (1996). Family-based treatment for adolescent problem behaviors: Overview of contemporary developments and introduction to the special section. *Journal of Family Psychology, 10,* 3–11.

Linehan, M. M. (1993). *Cognitive-behavioral treatment of borderline personality disorder.* New York: Guilford Press.

Loeber, R., & Farrington, D. P. (1998). *Serious and violent juvenile offenders: Risk factors and successful interventions.* Thousand Oaks, CA: Sage.

Lowinson, J. H., Ruiz, P., Millman, R. B., & Langrod, J. G. (Eds.). (1997). *Substance abuse: A comprehensive textbook* (3rd ed.). Baltimore: Williams & Wilkins.

Luthar, S. L. (1999). *Poverty and children's adjustment.* Thousand Oaks, CA: Sage.

Luthar, S. L., & Suchman, N. E. (2000). Relational psychotherapy mothers' group: A developmentally informed intervention for at-risk mothers. *Development and Psychopathology, 12,* 235–253.

March, J. S., & Leonard, H. L. (1996). Obsessive–compulsive disorder in children and adolescents: A review of the past 10 years. *Journal of the American Academy of Child and Adolescent Psychiatry, 34,* 1265–1272.

Maris, R. W. (1991). Introduction. *Suicide and Life-Threatening Behavior, 21,* 1–17.

Martin, W. E., & Swartz, J. L. (1997). Integrated application of applied ecological psychology in schools within communities. In J. L. Swartz & W. E. Martin (Eds.), *Applied ecological psychology for schools within communities* (pp. 209–220). Mahwah, NJ: Erlbaum.

Mash, E. J. (1998). Treatment of child and family disturbance: A behavioral–systems perspective. In E. J. Mash & R. A. Barkley (Eds.), *Treatment of childhood disorders* (2nd ed., pp. 3–51). New York: Guilford Press.

Mash, E. J., & Dozois, D. J. A. (1996). Child psychopathology: A developmental–systems perspective. In E. J. Mash & R. A. Barkley (Eds.), *Child psychopathology* (pp. 3–60). New York: Guilford Press.

Mayes, L. C., & Bornstein, M. H. (1997). The development of children exposed to cocaine. In S. S. Luthar, J. Burack, D. Cicchetti, & J. R. Weisz (Eds.), *Developmental psychopathology: Perspectives on adjustment, risk, and disorder* (pp. 166–188). New York: Cambridge University Press.

McBride, D. C., VanderWaal, C. J., Terry, Y. M., & VanBuren, H. (1999). *Breaking the cycle of drug use among juvenile offenders* (Publication No. NCJ 179273). Washington, DC: National Institute of Justice.

McClellan, J., & Werry, J. (1994). Practice parameters for the assessment and treatment of children and adolescents with schizophrenia. *Journal of the American Academy of Child and Adolescent Psychiatry, 33,* 616–635.

McDonald, T. P., Allen, R. I., Westerfelt, A., & Piliavin, I. (1996). *Assessing the long-term effects of foster care: A research synthesis.* Washington, DC: CWLA Press.

McEvoy, A., & Welker, R. (2001). Antisocial behavior, academic failure, and school climate: A critical review. In H. M. Walker & M. H. Epstein (Eds.), *Making schools safer and violence free: Critical issues, solutions, and recommended practices. A compilation of articles from the* Journal of Emotional and Behavioral Disorders (pp. 28–38). Austin, TX: Pro-Ed.

Measham, T. J. (1995). The acute management of aggressive behavior in hospitalized children and adolescents. *Canadian Journal of Psychiatry, 40,* 330–336.

Meichenbaum, D., & Turk, D. C. (1987). *Facilitating treatment adherence: A practitioner's guidebook.* New York: Plenum Press.

Melton, G. B., Petrila, J., Poythress, N. G., & Slobogin, C. (1997). *Psychological evaluations for the courts: A handbook for mental health professionals and lawyers* (2nd ed.). New York: Guilford Press.

Miller, M. L. (1998). *The Multisystemic Therapy Pilot Program: Final evaluation.* Wilmington, DE: Evaluation, Research, and Planning.

Minuchin, S. (1974). *Families and family therapy.* Cambridge, MA: Harvard University Press.

Monahan, J. (1981a). *Predicting violent behavior: An assessment of clinical techniques.* Beverly Hills, CA: Sage.

Monahan, J. (1981b). *The clinical prediction of violent behavior: Crime and delinquency issues.* Washington, DC: U.S. Government Printing Office.

Multimodal Treatment Study for Children with ADHD Cooperative Group. (1999). A 14–month randomized clinical trial of treatment strategies for attention deficit/hyperactivity disorder. *Archives of General Psychiatry, 56,* 1073–1086.

Munger, R. L. (1993). *Changing children's behavior quickly.* Lanham, MD: Madison Books.

National Institute on Drug Abuse. (1999). *Principles of drug addiction treatment: A research-based guide* (NIH Publication No. 99–4180). Rockville, MD: National Institutes of Health.

Nelson, K. E., & Landsman, M. J. (1992). *Alternative models of family preservation: Family-based services in context.* Springfield, IL: Thomas.

Ninan, P. T., & Mance, R. (1990). Schizophrenia and other psychotic disorders. In A.

Stoudemire (Ed.), *Clinical psychiatry for medical students* (pp. 107–136). Philadelphia: Lippincott.

Ogden, T. (2001). *Updating the Norwegian MST clinical trial.* Oslo: Center for Research in Clinical Psychology, Department of Psychology, University of Oslo.

O'Leary, K. D., Heyman, R. E., & Neidig, P. H. (1999). Treatment of wife abuse: A comparison of gender-specific and conjoint approaches. *Behavior Therapy, 30,* 475–507.

Ollendick, T. H., & King, N. J. (1998). Empirically supported treatments for children with phobic and anxiety disorders: Current status. *Journal of Clinical Child Psychology, 27,* 156–167.

Parke, R. D., O'Neil, R., Isley, S., Spitzer, S., Welsh, M., Wang, S., Flyr, M., Simpkins, S., Strand, C., & Morales, M. (1998). Family–peer relationships: Cognitive, emotional, and ecological determinants. In M. Lewis & C. Feiring (Eds.), *Families, risk, and competence* (pp. 89–112). Mahwah, NJ: Erlbaum.

Patterson, G. R. (1982). *Coercive family process.* Eugene, OR: Castalia.

Patterson, G. R. (1997). Performance models for parenting: A social interactional perspective. In J. E. Grusec & L. Kuczynski (Eds.), *Parenting and children's internalization of values: A handbook of contemporary theory* (pp. 193–226). New York: Wiley.

Patterson, G. R., & Reid, J. B. (1984). Social interactional processes in the family: The study of the moment by moment family transactions in which human social development is embedded. *Journal of Applied Developmental Psychology, 5,* 237–262.

Pettit, G. S., & Clawson, M. A. (1995). Pathways to interpersonal competence: Parenting and children's peer relations. In N. Vanzetti & S. Duck (Eds.), *A lifetime of relationships* (pp. 125–154). Pacific Grove, CA: Brooks/Cole.

Pfeffer, C. R., Klerman, G. L., Hurt, S. W., Lesser, M., Peskin, J. R., & Siefker, M. A. (1991). Suicidal children grow up: Demographic and clinical risk factors for adolescent suicide attempts. *Journal of the American Academy of Child and Adolescent Psychiatry, 30,* 609–616.

Pfefferbaum, B. (1997). Posttraumatic stress disorder in children: A review of the past 10 years. *Journal of the American Academy of Child and Adolescent Psychiatry, 36,* 1503–1511.

Pierce, G. R., Sarason, B. R., & Sarason, I. (1995). *Handbook of social support and the family.* New York: Plenum Press.

Pliszka, S. R., Carlson, C. L., & Swanson, J. M. (1999). *ADHD with comorbid disorders: Clinical assessment and management.* New York: Guilford Press.

Pliszka, S. R., Greenhill, L. L., Crismon, M. L., Sedillo, A., Carlson, C., Conners, C. K., McCracken, J. T., Swanson, J. M., Hughes, C. W., Llana, M. E., Lopez, M., & Toprac, M. G. (2000a). The Texas Children's Medication Algorithm Project: Report of the Texas Consensus Conference Panel on Medication Treatment of Childhood Attention-Deficit/Hyperactivity Disorder, Part I. *Journal of the American Academy of Child and Adolescent Psychiatry 39,* 908–919.

Pliszka, S. R., Greenhill, L. L., Crismon, M. L., Sedillo, A., Carlson, C., Conners, C. K., McCracken, J. T., Swanson, J. M., Hughes, C. W., Llana, M. E., Lopez, M., & Toprac, M. G. (2000b). The Texas Children's Medication Algorithm Project: Report of the Texas Consensus Conference Panel on Medication Treatment of Childhood Attention-Deficit/Hyperactivity Disorder, Part II. Tactics. *Journal of the American Academy of Child and Adolescent Psychiatry 39,* 920–927.

Poulin, F., Dishion, T. J., & Haas, E. (1999). The peer influence paradox: Friendship quality and deviancy training within adolescent male friendships. *Merrill–Palmer Quarterly, 45,* 42–61.

Quick, J. D., Nelson, D. L., Matuszek, P. A., Whittington, J. L., & Quick, J. C. (1996). Social support, secure attachments, and health. In C. L. Cooper (Ed.), *Handbook for stress, medicine, and health* (pp. 269–287). Boca Raton, FL: CRC Press.

Quiggle, N. L., Garber, J., Panak, W. F., & Dodge, K. A. (1992). Social information processing in aggressive and depressed children. *Child Development, 63,* 1305–1320.

Quinn, M. M., Kavale, K. A., Mathur, S. R., Rutherford, R. B., & Forness, S. R. (1999). A meta-analysis of social skills interventions for students with emotional or behavioral disorders. *Journal of Emotional and Behavioral Disorders, 7,* 54–64.

Quinsey, V. L., & Maguire, A. (1986). Maximum security psychiatric patients: Actuarial and clinical prediction of dangerousness. *Journal of Interpersonal Violence, 1,* 143–172.

Randall, J., Swenson, C. C., & Henggeler, S. W. (1999). Neighborhood Solutions for Neighborhood Problems: An empirically-based violence prevention collaboration. *Health, Education, and Behavior, 26,* 806–820.

Reinecke, M. A., Ryan, N. E., & DuBois, D. L. (1998). Cognitive-behavioral therapy of depression and depressive symptoms during adolescence: A review and meta-analysis. *Journal of the American Academy of Child and Adolescent Psychiatry, 37,* 26–34.

Reiss, D., & Price, R. H. (1996). National research agenda for prevention research: The National Institute of Mental Health report. *American Psychologist, 51,* 1109–1115.

Resnick, M., & Burton, B. T. (1984). Droperidol versus haloperidol in the initial management of acutely agitated patients. *Journal of Clinical Psychiatry, 45,* 298–299.

Rife, J., & Belcher, J. (1994). Assisting unemployed older workers become reemployed: An experimental evaluation. *Research on Social Work Practice, 4,* 3–13.

Rimmerman, A., Kramer, R., Levy, J. M., & Levy, P. H. (1989). Who benefits most from respite care? *International Journal of Rehabilitation Research, 12,* 41–47.

Rivera, V. R., & Kutash, K. (1994). *Components of a system of care: What does the research say?* Tampa: Research and Training Center for Children's Mental Health, Florida Mental Health Institute, University of South Florida.

Robin, A. L., Bedway, M., & Gilroy, M. (1994). Problem-solving communication training. In C. W. LeCroy (Ed.), *Handbook of child and adolescent treatment manuals* (pp. 92–124). New York: Lexington Books.

Rothbaum, B. O., Meadows, E. A., Resick, P., & Foy, D. W. (2000). Cognitive-behavioral therapy. In E. B. Foa, T. M., Keane, & M. J. Friedman (Eds.), *Effective treatments for PTSD: Practice guidelines from the International Society for Traumatic Stress Studies* (pp. 320–325). New York: Guilford Press.

Rowland, M. D., Cunningham, P. B., & Kruesi, M. (2001). *MST crisis safety checklists.* Unpublished instrument, Family Services Research Center, Department of Psychiatry and Behavioral Sciences, Medical University of South Carolina, Charleston.

Rowland, M. D., Halliday-Boykins, C. A., Henggeler, S. W., Cunningham, P. B., Lee, T. G., Donkervoet, J., Kruesi, M., & Shapiro, S. B. (2002). *A randomized trial of multisystemic therapy (MST) with Hawaii's Felix Class youth.* Manuscript submitted for publication.

Rowland, M. D., Henggeler, S. W., Gordon, A. M., Pickrel, S. G., Cunningham, P. B., & Edwards, J. E. (2000). Adapting multisystemic therapy to serve youth presenting psychiatric emergencies: Two case studies. *Child Psychology and Psychiatry Review, 5,* 30–43.

Rush, A. J., Crimson, M. L., Toprac, M., Trivedi, M. H., Rago, W. V., Shon, S., & Altshuler, K. Z. (1998). Consensus guidelines in the treatment of major depressive disorder. *Journal of Clinical Psychiatry, 59*(Suppl. 20), 73–84.

Salisbury, C. L., & Intagliata, J. (1986). *Respite care: Support for persons with developmental disabilities and their families.* Baltimore: Brookes.

Santos, A. B. (1996). Assertive community treatment. In S. Soreff (Ed.), *The seriously and persistently mentally ill: The state of the art treatment handbook* (pp. 411–431). Seattle: Hogrefe & Huber.

Satin, R. (2000). *A test of the efficacy of multisystemic therapy for reducing recidivism and decreasing the length of residential treatment.* Paper presented at the First Annual International MST Conference, Savannah, GA.

Sattler, J. (1992). Assessment of children's intelligence. In C. E. Walker & M. C. Roberts (Eds.), *Handbook of clinical child psychology* (2nd ed., pp. 85–100). New York: Wiley.

Schoenwald, S. K. (1998). *Multisystemic therapy consultation guidelines.* Charleston, SC: MST Institute.

Schoenwald, S. K. (2000, October). Transportability of new treatments: MST as a test case. In K. Hoagwood (Chair), *Taking effective treatments to scale: Research on service implementation.* Seminar presented at the annual meeting of the American Academy of Child and Adolescent Psychiatry, New York, NY.

Schoenwald, S. K., & Henggeler, S. W. (2002). Services research and family based treatment. In H. A. Liddle, D. A. Santisteban, R. F. Levant, & J. H. Bray (Eds.), *Family psychology: Science-based interventions* (pp. 259–282). Washington, DC: American Psychological Association.

Schoenwald, S. K., Henggeler, S. W., Brondino, M. J., & Rowland, M. D. (2000). Multisystemic therapy: Monitoring treatment fidelity. *Family Process, 39,* 83–103.

Schoenwald, S. K., Henggeler, S. W., & Edwards, D. (1998). *MST Supervisor Adherence Measure.* Charleston, SC: MST Institute.

Schoenwald, S. K., Ward, D. M., Henggeler, S. W., Pickrel, S. G., & Patel, H. (1996). MST treatment of substance abusing or dependent adolescent offenders: Costs of reducing incarceration, inpatient, and residential placement. *Journal of Child and Family Studies, 5,* 431–444.

Schoenwald, S. K., Ward, D. M., Henggeler, S. W., & Rowland, M. D. (2000). MST vs. hospitalization for crisis stabilization of youth: Placement outcomes 4 months post-referral. *Mental Health Services Research, 2,* 3–12.

Shores, R. E., & Wehby, J. H. (1999). Analyzing the classroom social behavior of students with EBD. *Journal of Emotional and Behavioral Disorders, 7,* 194–199.

Smith, K., Conroy, R. W., & Ehler, R. (1984). Lethality of Suicide Attempt Rating Scale. *Suicide and Life-Threatening Behavior, 14,* 215–242.

Spencer, E. K., Kafantaris, V., Padron-Gayol, M. V., Rosenberg, C. R., & Campbell, M. (1992). Haloperidol in schizophrenic children: Early findings from a study in progress. *Psychopharmacology Bulletin, 28,* 183–186.

Stanton, M. D., & Shadish, W. R. (1997). Outcome, attrition, and family-couples treatment for drug abuse: A meta-analysis and review of the controlled, comparative studies. *Psychological Bulletin, 122,* 170–191.

Stark, M. J. (1992). Dropping out of substance abuse treatment: A clinically oriented review. *Clinical Psychology Review, 12,* 93–116.

Steinberg, L., Lamborn, S., Darling, N., Mounts, N., & Dornbusch, S. (1994). Overtime changes in adjustment and competence among adolescents from authoritative, authoritarian, indulgent, and neglectful families. *Child Development, 65,* 754–770.

Strother, K. B., Swenson, M. E., & Schoenwald, S. K. (1998). *Multisystemic therapy organizational manual.* Charleston, SC: MST Institute.

Stroul, B. A. (1988) *Series on community-based services for children and adolescents who are severely emotionally disturbed, Vol. 1. Home-based services.* Washington, DC: CASSP Technical Assistance Center, Georgetown University Child Development Center.

Stroul, B. A., & Friedman, R. M. (1986). *A system of care for severely emotionally disturbed children and youth.* Washington, DC: Georgetown University Child Development Center.

Stroul, B. A., & Friedman, R. M. (1996). *A system of care for children and adolescents with severe emotional disturbance* (Rev. ed.). Washington, DC: National Technical Assistance Center for Child Mental Health, Georgetown University Child Development Center.

Tate, D. C., Reppucci, N. D., & Mulvey, E. P. (1995). Violent juvenile delinquents: Treatment effectiveness and implications for future action. *American Psychologist, 50,* 777–781.

Thomas, C. R., Holzer, C. E., & Wall, J. (2002). The Island Youth Programs: Community interventions for reducing youth violence and delinquency. *Adolescent Psychiatry: The Annals of the American Society for Adolescent Psychiatry, 26,* 125–143.

Thomas, H., Jr., Schwartz, E., & Petrilli, R. (1992). Droperidol versus haloperidol for chemical restraint of agitated and combative patients. *Annals of Emergency Medicine, 21,* 407–413.

Tolbert, H. A. (1996). Psychosis in children and adolescents: A review. *Journal of Clinical Psychiatry, 57*(Suppl. 3), 4–8.

Tomb, D. A. (1995). *Psychiatry for the house officer.* Baltimore: Williams & Wilkins.

Torrey, E. F. (1988). *Surviving schizophrenia: A family manual.* New York: Harper & Row.

Trickett, E. J. (1997). Developing an ecological mind-set on school–community collaboration. In J. L. Swartz & W. E. Martin (Eds.), *Applied ecological psychology for schools within communities* (pp. 139–166). Mahwah, NJ: Erlbaum.

Unger, D. G., & Wandersman, A. (1985). The importance of neighbors: The social, cognitive, and affective components of neighboring. *American Journal of Community Psychology, 13,* 139–169.

Upshur, C. C. (1982a). Respite care for mentally retarded and other disabled populations: Program models and family needs. *Mental Retardation, 20,* 2–6.

Upshur, C. C. (1982b). An evaluation of home-based respite care. *Mental Retardation, 20,* 58–62.

U.S. Bureau of the Census. (1995). Marital status and living arrangements, March 1995 (Update). *Current Population Reports* (P20–491). Washington, DC: U.S. Government Printing Office.

U.S. Department of Health and Human Services. (1999). *Mental health: A report of the Surgeon General.* Rockville, MD: National Institute of Mental Health, National Institutes of Health, U.S. Department of Health and Human Services.

U.S. Public Health Service. (2000). *Report of the Surgeon General's Conference on Children's Mental Health: A national action agenda.* Washington, DC: Author.

U.S. Public Health Service. (2001). *Youth violence: A report of the Surgeon General.* Washington, DC: Author.

Vaughn, C. E., & Leff, J. P. (1976). The influence of family and social factors on the course of psychiatric illnesses: A comparison of schizophrenic and depressed neurotic patients. *British Journal of Psychiatry, 129,* 125–137.

Visher, E. B., & Visher, J. S. (1993). Remarriage families and stepparenting. In F. Walsh (Ed.) *Normal family processes* (2nd ed., pp. 235–253). New York: Guilford Press.

Volkmar, F. R. (1996). Child and adolescent psychosis: A review of the past 10 years. *Journal of the American Academy of Child and Adolescent Psychiatry, 35,* 843–851.

Wahler, R. G. (1980). The insular mother: Her problems in parent–child treatment. *Journal of Applied Behavior Analysis, 13,* 207–219.

Wahler, R. G. (1990). Some perceptual functions of social networks in coercive mother–child interactions. *Journal of Social and Clinical Psychology, 9,* 43–53.

Walker, H. M., & Epstein, M. H. (Eds.). (2001). *Making schools safer and violence free: Critical issues, solutions, and recommended practices.* Austin, TX: Pro-Ed.

Walker, H. M., Horner, R. H., Sugai, G., Bullis, M., Sprague, J. R., Bricker, D., & Kauffman, M. J. (1996). Integrated approaches to preventing antisocial behavior patterns among school-age children and youth. *Journal of Emotional and Behavioral Disorders, 4,* 194–209.

Warren, R., & Cohen, S. (1985). Respite care. *Rehabilitation Literature, 46,* 66–71.

Washington State Institute for Public Policy. (1998). *Watching the bottom line: Cost-effective interventions for reducing crime in Washington.* Olympia, WA: Evergreen State College.

Webster-Stratton, C. (1998). Preventing conduct problems in Head Start children: Strengthening parent competencies. *Journal of Consulting and Clinical Psychology, 66,* 715–730.

Webster-Stratton, C., & Hammond, M. (1997). Treating children with early-onset conduct problems: A comparison of child and parent training interventions. *Journal of Consulting and Clinical Psychology, 65,* 93–109.

Webster-Stratton, C., & Herbert, M. (1994). *Troubled families: Problem children.* New York: Wiley.

Wechsler, D. (1991). *Manual for the Wechsler Intelligence Scale for Children* (3rd ed.). San Antonio, TX: Psychological Corporation.

Wehby, J. H., Symons, F. J., & Shores, R. E. (1995). A descriptive analysis of aggressive behavior in classrooms for children with emotional and behavioral disorders. *Behavioral Disorders, 20,* 87–105.

Weiss, B., Catron, T., & Harris, V. (2001). *Independent evaluation of the MST services package.* Nashville, TN: Center for Psychotherapy Research and Policy, Vanderbilt University.

Weisz, J. R., Han, S. S., & Valeri, S. M. (1997). More of what?: Issues raised by the Fort Bragg Study. *American Psychologist, 52,* 541–545.

Weisz, J. R., & Jensen, P. S. (1999). Efficacy and effectiveness of child and adolescent psychotherapy and pharmacotherapy. *Mental Health Services Research, 1,* 125–157.

Xie, H., Cairns, R. B., & Cairns, B. D. (1999). Social networks and configurations in inner-city schools: Aggression, popularity, and implications for students with EBD. *Journal of Emotional and Behavioral Disorders, 7,* 147–155.

Zealberg, J. J., Finkenbine, R., & Christie, S. (1995). *An overview of emergency psychopharmacology.* Unpublished manuscript, Department of Psychiatry and Behavioral Sciences, Medical University of South Carolina, Charleston.

# Index

"f" indicates a figure; "t" indicates a table

Academic testing, 83
Accountability, 8–9, 28
Affective bonding, 59–61
Alcohol abuse. *See* Substance abuse
Analytic process. *See* MST analytic process
Annie E. Casey Foundation, 141
Antisocial behavior, 5, 12, 109
Anxiety disorders, 13, 54–55
Appraisal support, 70
Assertive community treatment, 55
Assessments
    family resource specialists and, 144–145
    of peer relations, 88–89
    respite care and, 150–151
    of service ecology, 75–76
    therapeutic foster care and, 158–159
    *See also* Crisis assessment; Family
        assessments; Fit assessments; Intake
        assessments; School assessments
Attention-deficit/hyperactivity disorder
    (ADHD), 14–15
Authoritarian parenting, 40–41
Authoritative parenting, 40

Bipolar disorder, 13

Caregivers. *See* Parents/caregivers
Childhood depression, 109
Child physical abuse, 218
Clinical support, 9–10
Cognitive-behavioral therapy (CBT), 7, 14
Collaborative working relationships, 150
Command–compliance interactions, 175–176

Commitments, 135–136
Communities
    evaluating in crisis assessments, 125
    MST transportability studies, 221
    school–community linkage, 82
Conflict resolution strategies, 94
Consultants, 231
Coparenting relationships
    interventions for, 61–69
    risk factors for child behavior problems,
        41–43
Criminal behavior, MST outcomes for, 210–
    212
Crises
    defined, 99–100
    MST outcomes for, 209–210
    predictable and unpredictable, 103–108
    risk factors, 127t
Crisis assessment
    family and immediate social environment,
        118–119
    home/living environment, 119, 123–124
    homicidal youths, 111–113
    neighborhoods and communities, 125
    peer relations, 124–125
    psychotic behavior, 115–118
    risk factors for serious emotional
        disturbances, 108–111
    Safety Checklist, 120–123f
    suicidal youths, 113–115
Crisis Assessment of Youth, Family, and
    Environment Form, 126, 128f
Crisis caseworkers, 102–103

Crisis interventions
crisis teams, 100–103
goals of, 99–100
integrating risk factors to determine
placement site, 125–130
predictable and unpredictable crises, 103–
108
Crisis management
behavioral interventions, 131–133
commitments, 135–136
elements of, 130–131
guidelines for interacting with other
agencies and professionals, 137–138
MST principles in, 131
overview of, 102–103
police interventions, 136–137
psychopharmacological interventions,
133–134
therapeutic holds, 134–135
Crisis Safety Checklist, 120–123f
Crisis Safety Plan Form, 132, 133f
Crisis teams
administrators, 100–101
child psychiatrists, 103
client safety and, 108
crisis caseworkers, 102–103
crisis management procedures, 130–131
integrating responsibilities, 103–108
purpose and overview of, 100
response to predictable crises, 104–106
response to unpredictable crises, 107–108
Safety Plan Form, 132, 133f
supervisors, 101–102
therapists, 102

Delaware Alternative to Secure Care Project,
214–215
Delirium, 116
Delusions, 115–116
Dementia, 116
Depression, 12, 53–54, 55, 109
Deviancy training, 80–81, 87, 177
Diabetes, 224
Discipline strategies, changing, 45–46
Divorced parents, interventions for, 66–67

Emergency commitment, 135
Emotional support, 70
Engagement
case example, 178
defined, 150
respite care and, 150
therapeutic foster care and, 158
Estranged parents, interventions for, 66–67
Evaluations, 28. See also Assessments
Evidence-based interventions, 7
Expert consultations, 231
Extinction and extinction bursts, 132

Families
crisis treatment plans and, 129
empowerment of, 28–29
family–school linkage, 81–82
forms of, 38

functions of, 38–39
increasing social support for, 70–73, 145–
147
in peer interventions, 92–93
peer relations of children and, 88
risk and protective factors, 44
in school-related interventions, 86–87
systems perspective, 39–40
Family assessments, 118–119
case example, 175–176
Family functioning
MST outcome studies, 209
school-related problems and, 82–83
Family interventions
addressing barriers to effective parenting
practices, 49–61
anticipating child's testing of parenting
practices, 48–49
case examples, 178–180, 189–190, 198–
199
changing parenting practices, 45–47
diversity of treatment targets and clinical
competencies, 73–74
enlisting support of caregivers, 44–45
implementation of new parenting
practices, 49
increasing social support, 70–73
monitoring youth behavior, 46–47
preparing caregivers for negative child
reactions, 47–48
protective factors identified, 44
risk factors identified, 39–43
Family resource specialists (FRS), 143–148
Family risk factors
individual caregiver factors, 43
parenting practices, 40–41
relations among coparents, 41–43
systems perspective, 39–40
Family Services Research Center, 141
Firearms, 111, 123–124
"Fit analysis," 30–31
Fit assessments
case examples, 174–177, 186–188, 195–
197
descriptions of, 22–24, 30–31
"Fit circles," 31
Foster care. See Therapeutic foster care (TFC)

Hallucinations, 115
Healthy Children Through Healthy Schools
project, 220
Home-based service delivery, 6–7, 35–36
therapeutic foster care and, 154–156
Home/living environment
crisis assessment and, 119, 123–124
crisis treatment plans and, 129–130
Homicidal youths, 111–113, 124
Hospital placements. See Psychiatric
inpatient placements
Hypothesis development and testing, 31–33

Incarceration, MST outcomes for, 210–212
Informal social support, 146
Information support, 70

Instrumental support, 70
Insulin-dependent diabetes mellitus, 224
Intake assessments, case examples, 170–171,
    184–186, 193–195
Intelligence, school-related problems and, 83
Intelligence testing, 83
Intermediary goals, 33, 35
Island Youth Programs, 216

Judicial commitment, 135–136
Juvenile drug courts, 218–219
Juvenile sexual offenders, 215–216

Learning disabilities, school-related problems
    and, 83
Living environment. See Home/living
    environment

Marital interventions
    changing instrumental relations, 64–65
    clarifying parental roles, 69
    dealing with negative affect, 62–64
    dealing with physical abuse, 65–66
    for divorced or estranged parents, 66–67
    general features of, 61
    setting the stage for, 61–62
    stepfamily adjustments, 67–69
Marital violence, 65–66
Mental health problems
    MST outcome studies, 208–210
    risk factors, 108–111
    role of MST in treating, 10–16
    social-ecological view of, 12–15
    Surgeon General's report on and action
        agenda for, 11–12, 224–226
Monitoring, 46–47, 124
MST. See Multisystemic therapy
MST analytic process, 18
    clarifying reasons for referrals, 29–30
    developing overarching goals, 30
    hypothesis development and testing, 31–
        33
    identifying and overcoming barriers to
        progress, 34–35
    intermediary treatment goals, 33, 35
    intervention development and
        implementation, 33–34
MST-based continuum of care
    basis and origins of, 139–141
    family resource specialists, 143–148
    key features of, 141–142
    ongoing research projects, 219–220
    psychopharmacological interventions,
        166–167
    purpose of, 141
    residential and psychiatric inpatient
        placements, 162–166
    respite care, 148–154
    service delivery models, 142
    therapeutic foster care, 154–162
"MST Do-Loop," 18, 29
MST interventions
    case examples, 180–181, 190–191, 198
    development and implementation, 33–34

developmental appropriateness, 27
empowerment of families and caregivers,
    28–29
evaluation and accountability, 28
evidence-based, 7
finding and understanding fit factors, 22–
    24
identifying and overcoming barriers, 34–
    35
increasing responsible behavior, 25–26
need for continual effort in, 27–28
present-focused, action-oriented, 26
targeting sequences of behavior, 26–27
treatment principles, 19–22
using strengths as levers for change, 24–
    25
See also Crisis interventions; Family
    interventions; Marital interventions;
    Peer interventions; School-related
    interventions
MST outcomes
    for criminal behavior and violence, 210–
        212
    Delaware Alternative to Secure Care
        Project trial, 214–215
    identifying and measuring, 232–233
    Island Youth Programs, 216
    juvenile sexual offender replication trial,
        215–216
    for mental health problems, 208–210
    Ontario multisite trial, 215
    overview of studies, 206–208, 217
    for substance abuse and dependence, 212–
        214
MST quality assurance, 9–10
    continuous quality improvement system,
        234–239
    internal capacity building, 239–240
    manualization of program components,
        229–231
    MST training package, 231–234
    overview of, 228–229
    purpose of, 228
    rationale for, 227–228
MST research
    Healthy Children Through Healthy
        Schools project, 220
    on juvenile drug courts, 218–219
    on MST-based continuum of care, 219–220
    Neighborhood Solutions for Neighborhood
        Problems project, 220
    New York multisite clinical trial, 222–223
    Norwegian multisite clinical trial, 221–
        222
    on physically abused children, 218
    Stark County Mental Health Board, Ohio,
        223
    transportability studies, 221
    Vanderbilt University, 223
    Washington state multisite clinical trial,
        222
    Wayne State University, Children's
        Hospital, 224
MST training package, 231–234

Multisystemic therapy (MST), 3–4
 adapting for youths with serious
  emotional disturbances, 97–98
 case examples, 169–183, 183–192, 192–
  200
 conditions when indicated, 15
 conditions when not indicated, 16
 least restrictive environment philosophy
  and, 162–163
 limitations of traditional programs, 139–
  140
 privileges and challenges to therapists,
  17–18
 role in treating mental health problems,
  10–16
 treatment principles, 19–22

Neglectful parenting, 41
Neighborhoods
 crisis treatment plans and, 129–130
 evaluating in crisis assessments, 125
Neighborhood Solutions for Neighborhood
  Problems project, 220
Neuroleptics, 117
New York multisite clinical trial, 222–223
Norway
 MST capacity building, 239–240
 multisite clinical trials, 221–222

Obsessive–compulsive disorder (OCD), 13–
  14
Ohio
 MST capacity building, 240
 MST research studies, 223
Ontario multisite trial, 215
Organizational support, 231
Outcomes. See MST outcomes
Overarching goals. See Treatment goals

Parenting practices
 addressing barriers to successful child
  outcomes, 49–61
 anticipating child's testing of, 48–49
 changing with family interventions, 45–47
 child characteristics and, 58–59
 effects of parental knowledge and skills
  on child outcomes, 49–52
 implementation of new practices, 49
 low affective bonding and, 59–61
 parental mental health problems and, 52–
  56
 parental substance abuse and, 56–57
 practical challenges, 57–58
 risk factors for child behavior problems,
  40, 41
 social supports, 44
 types of, 40–41
Parents/caregivers
 clarifying parental roles, 69
 effects of knowledge and skills on child
  outcomes, 49–52
 empowerment of, 28–29
 enlisting support of, 44–45
 low affective bonding and, 59–61

mental health problems and, 52–56
 monitoring youth behavior, 46–47
 in MST programs, 7–8
 in peer interventions, 90–92
 peer relations of children and, 88
 preparing for negative child reactions, 47–
  48
 risk factors for child behavior problems,
  40, 41, 43
 in school-related interventions, 86–87
 substance abuse and, 56–57
Peer interventions
 case examples, 199–200
 changing peer affiliations, 89–90
 family involvement in, 92–93
 role of caregivers in, 90–92
 targeting social problem-solving skills, 94–
  95
Peer relations
 assessing and understanding, 80–81, 88–
  89
 cognitive-behavioral interventions and,
  93
 crisis treatment plans and, 129–130
 evaluating in crisis assessments, 124–125
 overcoming peer neglect/rejection, 92
 significance of, 87–88
Permissive parenting, 41
Physical abuse. See Child physical abuse;
  Marital violence
Police, in crisis management, 136–137
Posttraumatic stress disorder (PTSD), 14,
  54–55
Predictable crises, 103–106
Privileges, 46
Problem-solving interventions, for social
  skills, 94–95
Protective factors, 6, 44
Proximal causes, 32
Psychiatric emergencies. See Crises
Psychiatric inpatient placements, 162–166
Psychiatrists, 103, 164, 166–167
Psychopharmacological interventions, 133–
  134, 166–167, 190–191
Psychotic behavior, 55
 crisis assessment, 115–118
 environmental factors and, 117
 medical conditions and, 116–117
 medication and, 117
 risk factors among adolescents, 109–110
Punishers, 132

Quality assurance. See MST quality
  assurance

Rearrests, MST outcomes for, 210–212
Referrals, clarifying reasons for, 29–30
Reinforcers, 132
Residential placements, 162–165
Respite care, 148
 appropriate uses, 149–151
 objectives of, 148–149
 providers, 151–152
 therapist responsibilities in, 152–154

Responsibility, increasing behavior for, 25–
        26
Risk factors
    addressed by multisystemic therapy, 5–6
    for adolescent psychosis, 109–110
    for adolescent suicide, 110–111
    for antisocial behavior, 5, 109
    for childhood depression, 109
    crisis treatment plan development and,
        125–130
    for psychiatric emergencies, 127t
    See also Family risk factors
Rules, 46

Safety Plan Form, 132, 133f
Safety plans
    case examples, 173–174, 188–189, 195
    therapeutic foster care and, 157–158
Schizophrenia, 55
School assessments, 79–83, 81, 176–177
School attendance, MST outcomes for, 209
School-related interventions
    assessing and understanding school-related
        problems, 79–83
    case examples, 181–183, 200
    engaging school personnel, 83–85
    establishing common goals, 85–86
    role of families and caregivers in, 86–87
School-related problems, assessing and
        understanding, 79–83
Service delivery
    home-based, 6–7, 35–36
    for MST-based continuum of care, 142
Service system interventions, 75–79
Social ecology/environment
    crisis assessment and, 118–119
    crisis treatment plans and, 129
    mental health problems and, 12–15
Social skills interventions, 94–95
Social support, 44
    assessing, 70–71
    case examples, 190
    developing, 71–73
    facilitating access to, 146–147
    importance of, 145–146
    for managing predictable crises, 105–106
    types of, 70
Stark County Mental Health Board, Ohio,
        223
Stepfamilies, 67–69
Strengths, using as levers for change, 24–25

Substance abuse, 56–57, 212–214
Substance intoxication, 116–117
Suicide, 110–111, 113–115, 124
Supervision, overview of, 229–230
Supervisor Adherence Measure, 235, 237–
        238t, 239

Teacher–student interactions, 80
Therapeutic foster care (TFC)
    case example, 161–162
    goals of, 154
    as an intervention, 160
    MST home-based care and, 154–156
    MST treatment goals and, 158–161
    tasks to be accomplished during, 156–158
Therapeutic holds, 134–135
Therapist Adherence Measure, 235, 236t
Thought disorders, 116
Training. See MST training package
Treatment barriers
    addressing barriers to effective parenting
        practices, 49–61
    family resource specialists and, 147
    identifying and overcoming, 34–35
    respite care and, 151
    using therapeutic foster care to address,
        160–161
Treatment goals
    case examples, 177–178, 188, 197–198
    developing, 30
    establishing in school-related
        interventions, 85–86
    intermediary, 33, 35
    problems with intervention success and,
        35
Treatment manuals, 229–230
Treatment sessions, 36
Treatment specification, 19

U.S. Surgeon General, 11–12, 224–226
Unpredictable crises, 104, 107–108

Vanderbilt University, 223
Violent behavior, MST outcomes for, 210–
        212

Washington state multisite clinical trial, 222
Wayne State University, Children's Hospital,
        224
Weapons, crisis assessments and, 123–124
Withdrawal, psychotic behavior and, 117